FOOD THERAPY

THE ULTIMATE GUIDE
TO CONSCIOUS EATING

MARLENE LASZLO, MSW

A SOLUTION GUIDE
FRIDAY PUBLISHING

COPYRIGHT © 2013
BY MARLENE LASZLO.

FridayPublishing@gmail.com
Marlene Laszlo/Friday Publishing
British Columbia, Canada

Food Therapy/ Marlene Laszlo. —1st ed.
ISBN 978-0-9881369-3-9

FOR THE WOMAN WHO
LOVES TO EAT,
LACKS WILLPOWER,
YET STILL WANTS TO
LOOK AND FEEL GREAT
AT ANY AGE

WE ARE FREE UP TO THE POINT OF CHOICE.
THEN THE CHOICE CONTROLS THE CHOOSER.

—Mary Crowley

Acknowledgements

I would like to thank Judy Hall, my "Lake Chapala" friend, for her inspiration and support during times when I felt stuck. A special thanks, too, to my son Chris for his ongoing encouragement, and a sincere thanks to my sister, Jeanette, for her insightful comments and ideas.

I'd also like to thank Nancy Adams for her thorough copyedit of the manuscript. As I did not always incorporate her changes, any errors that remain are mine.

Contents

OPEN THE DOOR TO POSSIBILITY 11

UNCOMMON SENSE WISDOM 17

Five Uncommon Sense Concepts....................................17

1. Say Hello To Your Other Self 18

2. Become More Superficial 21

3. Lower Your Expectations..23

4. Prepare For Failure 27

5. Expect Fear 29

THE POWER OF SMALL...31

In The "Now" 31

ILLUMINATE YOUR JOURNEY GOAL...........................39

The Success Secret 40

Decipher A Diet...41

DON'T BELIEVE EVERYTHING YOU THINK.............49

Your Learning Style...51

Contents

YOUR BUILT-IN COMPUTER 56

    How We Make Mindless Habits 58

    How Mindless Habits Can Work for You 60

THE HABIT-WILLPOWER CONNECTION 64

    How We Lose Willpower 66

    The Willpower Muscle 67

    Willpower Traps 69

    False Hope Trap 70

    "For Your Own Good" Trap 72

    "Fear of Self-Indulgence" Trap 73

    Escape From "Bad Feelings" Trap 74

    Getting Beyond The Traps 76

Contents

"GOOD INTENTION" MYTHS 78

Myth # 1 - I'm Investing In Myself 79

Myth # 2 - I Need To Spread the News 81

Myth # 3 - I'm Too Old 83

Myth # 4 - But I Have To Lose Weight First 85

Myth # 5 - Health Foods will Make Me Healthy 88

Myth # 6 - I Deserve A Treat 91

Myth # 7 - I'm Waiting for a Magic Remedy 92

FOOD TRAPS 95

Genetics Versus Biology 95

When Are You Full? 97

Warehouse Shopping Trap 99

Economy-Size Containers 100

Booby-Traps 102

Contents

The Convenience Trap 104

The "Crispy, Battered Nugget" Trap 106

THE FOOD THERAPY ADVANTAGE 108

Timing: When You Eat and What 108

Fuel Food 111

Savoring Food 115

Snacking Food 118

Luxury Food 122

Maintain Perspective 124

End Notes & Reminders 125

References 129

About the Author 133

CHAPTER 1

OPEN THE DOOR TO POSSIBILITY

The greatest challenge to any thinker is stating the problem in a way that will allow a solution.
— Bertrand Russell

When you utter the words "Food Therapy," how do you feel? Do you find the notion of being presented with food instead of talk a tempting concept? But what do I really mean by the words "*Food Therapy*"? Well, I chose this phrase because it best describes how I came to feel about the joy of eating after I learned how to get off the diet treadmill of guilty binges followed by dismal deprivation. For me—a true food lover—that was "therapy" with a very special twist.

FOOD THERAPY

At the same time, *Food Therapy* relates to the psychological aspects of our food choices. And with so many choices, our mental state is often embroiled in a battle between our rational and emotional sides. The problem with ignoring the psychological aspects of our food choices is that we think our rational side is in control when, really, our emotional side is in the driver's seat.

This book is about taking back control; about waking up your rational side so that you can make choices that work in your favor. Choices that not only satisfy your desire to indulge but also support your need to eat healthy and maintain a satisfactory weight.

Ellen Langer, author of the inspiring book, *Counter Clockwise: Mindful Health and the Power of Possibility,* offers the following words of wisdom: "The psychology of possibility first requires that we begin with the assumption that we do not know what we can do or become."

Are you ready to open the door to the possibilities in your life?

How I Started

> *"All the significant battles are waged within the self."*
> - Sheldon Kopp

By the time I was in my late twenties, I had been relying on dieting as my method of keeping the extra weight at bay for more than ten years. I lost and gained the same fifteen pounds over and over until I realized I was fighting a losing battle. A battle between my willpower and the tempting foods I knew I should not eat. All I wanted was to enjoy the social aspects and comfort that go along with eating and at

Dare to Explore "Foolish" Dreams

the same time maintain a reasonable weight; yet it seemed that the only way to have both was to alternate between "feast" and "famine." The notion that I could enjoy eating without either dieting or being overgrown seemed impossible.

overweight seemed impossible.

I secretly resented those "lucky ones" who, apparently, were able to eat whatever they wanted without gaining a pound. So I made a decision to come to grips with my body and accept myself the way I was. After all, the majority of people gain several pounds with each decade and, as my thirtieth birthday loomed, I told myself the extra weight was inevitable.

I made a decision to quit dieting. No more starvation, no more deprivation, no more foolish dreams of "having my cake and eating it too." It seemed a reasonable plan, and I held to it for several months—during which time I gained yet more weight. And I might have continued to accept this theory but for a small, serendipitous happening that goaded me out of my complacent choice.

A Serendipitous Surprise

"Alas! The fearful unbelief is unbelief in yourself."
- Thomas Carlyle

I was clearing out my closet, intending to discard the clothing I'd "outgrown," when I came across a pair of my favorite jeans. I held them up, recalling how good I used to feel when wearing them. The thought even crossed my mind that maybe I should try another diet. But I knew that was foolish thinking, and I reminded myself I was now into "self-acceptance." Closing my eyes, I tossed the jeans onto the growing heap.

A short while later I was getting the discards ready to be taken away when I had a sudden need to try on the jeans one last time. Wishful thinking, I knew, when I recalled that a few months before I could barely get them over my thighs. Nevertheless, I pulled off the elastic-waist sweats, which were now my comfortable attire, and stepped into my jeans, prepared for the tight squeeze. To my surprise, they went on without too much of a struggle.

Pay Special Attention To The Little Gifts

Perplexed, I walked over to the mirror, certain that I had made a mistake. Could they be the same jeans? Yet, as I studied my image, it was clear that they were the same. Still too snug—true—but the last time I couldn't even get them on. Which meant that something had happened to my body.

I scrutinized myself again in the mirror. I'd gotten rid of my scales, but from the fit of the jeans I'd obviously lost several pounds. How could that be? I was eating as usual, and I hadn't even thought of dieting for several months.

Glancing at the clock, I realized that I needed to hurry. I was preparing for exams at the university, where I'd enrolled as a mature student. Whatever had happened regarding my weight, I'd just have to chalk up to one of life's little miracles. A gift that I might as well enjoy while it lasted.

Think Like a Sleuth

That night, as was my habit before sleep, I was reading one of my favorite Sherlock Holmes mysteries. Holmes was talking to Watson and, throwing himself into an armchair, he said, "You see, but you do not observe. The distinction is clear."

His words resonated. I set down the book and contemplated my unexpected weight loss. I did see that I'd lost a few pounds. But could it be that I wasn't really using my powers of  observation? Was I missing the bigger picture, or the small details?

I was fearful of falling back into the trap of obsessing over my weight. Yet, what if I'd glimpsed a possibility that could really work? Maybe I needed to take the Sherlock Holmes approach: to not only see, but to observe what I'd been doing differently. If I figured this out, then perhaps I could use the information to guide me in the future.

With that thought, I turned off the light. Even in the darkness, I felt that a door had opened and a sliver of light was shining through. I was faced with a choice: Enter and discover what was on the other side, or chalk it up to coincidence and carry on as before.

As it turned out, I decided to open the door. Although I did not find one simple answer that miraculously changed my life overnight, my moment of insight started me on a different path. Instead of focusing so much on problems, I started to look at what was already working and then expanded on that.

As time went on and I completed my training as a psychotherapist, I continued to build my solution toolkit by combining my personal discoveries with relevant research and therapeutic techniques. In the process, I discovered that luck is something we cultivate from possibility rather than something that appears in full bloom.

Bite-Size Strategies

Dare to Enter And Discover

Food Therapy is a collection of bite-size strategies, related research, and personal tips that I have integrated over the years. It does not offer or promote any formal diet, but rather is designed to assist individuals in building a custom-made, personal toolkit. And although I cannot promise that reading this book will cause you to develop a wild craving for broccoli or a rigid resistance to chocolate, I can promise that these concepts worked for me and that they are open to anyone who chooses to use them.

> *Great things are not done by impulse, but by a series of small things brought together.*
> - **Vincent van Gogh**

CHAPTER 2

UNCOMMON SENSE WISDOM

There is nothing so unnatural as the commonplace.
-Sherlock Holmes

Five Uncommon Sense Concepts

The key factor that started my progression of change, as previously noted, was when I began to look at my challenge with different eyes. Instead of remaining stuck in the belief that there is only one way of looking at a dilemma—the common-sense way that everybody knows to be right—I allowed myself to consider diverse possibilities. Possibilities that weren't necessarily "common sense."

Become a Collector of Possibilities

As a result, I became a collector of "uncommon-sense" ideas, notions, and concepts, many, of which, I illustrate in this book. However, to get you thinking—and seeing—a bit differently, I will begin by introducing my top five that I hope will start you thinking beyond the obvious. Even if you don't agree with all of them, perhaps they will help you start to envision how many possibilities exist that we don't even consider.

1. Say Hello To Your Other Self

"If passion drives you, let reason hold the reins."
- Benjamin Franklin

Imagine this scenario: You walk into a fast food joint with the clear intention of ordering the salad until some-body walks by with a giant burger and fries. The clerk is ready to take your order. You glance up at the menu, at the picture of the salad you intend to order, then out of the blue you hear yourself say, "I'll have the king size burger." The clerk says, "With fries?" You hesitate, but only for a moment. "Sure. Make that a large."

Don't Underestimate the Power of Your Emotional Side

How does that happen? You walk in with your mind made up, yet, like the flip of an interior switch, your best-laid plans crumble and you walk out with triple the calories you intended. So what's going on here? The psychological explanation is that your emotional side—the thought process I sometimes refer to as the "Inner Con"—has outwrestled your rational side. In other words, you are of two minds.

Even though we know we have an emotional side—the side that makes us cry at sad movies or behave in ways that we later regret—we don't take that side too seriously. In spite of evidence to the contrary, most of us mindlessly take for granted that we can count on our cool, rational self to steer us in the right direction. In his book *The Happiness Hypothesis*, author Jonathan Haidt metaphorically describes the emotional side of our brain to be the size of an elephant and our rational side the size of a trainer.

> *"I am dragged along by a . . . strange force. Desire and reason are pulling in different directions.*
> *I see the right way and approve it but follow the wrong."*
> **-Ovid**
> **Metamorphoses**

What Size Are Your Emotions?

Years ago when I was backpacking in Southeast Asia, I decided that my experience would not be complete without going on an elephant trek. Right after signing up for the trek I read a newspaper article about an elephant that refused to obey its trainer and went on a wild rampage through a village.

The next day as I stood looking up at the massive creature, I realized it could easily crush me with one foot. I'd always thought of elephants as submissive circus creatures, but as I climbed the rope ladder I fully realized that my beliefs had been based in fantasy. In reality, the animal was powerful beyond my imagination, and I could only hope that the trainer was very adept.

Research bears out that we overestimate the power of our rational side—the trainer—and vastly underestimate the power of our emotions—our elephantine side. As much as we know that binge eating, overeating, comfort eating, and just plain bad eating are not rational decisions, we continue to believe that all we need do is exert enough self-control and the problem will go away. So one of the first steps in the change process is to give credit where credit is due. Don't underestimate the power of your emotional side.

- Are you aware of a struggle between your rational and emotional sides?
- Which side tends to win out more often when it comes to food choices?
- How do you feel when you give in to your emotional food cravings?

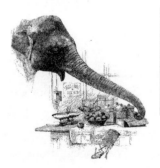

**I'LL EAT ALL
I WANT
TODAY AND DIET
TOMORROW**

2. Become More Superficial

"The first rule of holes: When you are in one,
stop digging."
                                        - Molly Ivins

What is your most common mode of operation when you feel that you have failed at the same thing over and over?

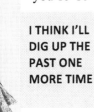

Do you ever reach a point where you're so frustrated that you decide there must be a deep-rooted reason buried in your past? If so, you're like most of us who, every once in awhile, decide we need to take a trip down memory lane to uncover the real root of why we keep repeating the same old habits.

I THINK I'LL DIG UP THE PAST ONE MORE TIME

The fact is, most of us have spent many hours speculating on the cause and reasons for a behavior, and often have come up with plenty of answers. But what does all that digging and all those answers really amount to?

You might notice a pattern of behavior that you can change, or, you might end up feeling frustrated like Sherry, in the following example:

The Deep-Rooted Trap

After long hours of analyzing her problem and reading self-help books, Sherry figured out that her habit of turning to food for comfort had started as a young girl. When her mother worked the evening shift and she had to stay alone, Sherry would be allowed to order a favorite treat such as pizza. Even though she felt lonely, the special treat comforted her. As an adult, even though she understood the root of her problem, she still could not figure out how to change her binge eating. She decided that this was a job for a professional. After spending many hours consulting with an expert, she discovered that not only was food a comfort, but that as a child she'd also learned to see food as a punishment (when she couldn't have dessert if she didn't eat the liver and onions). Food was also a reward for good behavior. Many sessions and dollars later, she had the information— food was reward, punishment, and comfort. Yet Sherry still didn't have an answer that would tell her how to stop her eating binges.

Where Are You Heading?

"If you do not change your direction, you will end up where you are heading"
- Confucius

The fact is that our rational side loves to contemplate and often gets more satisfaction out of analyzing than doing. Unfortunately, knowing "why" we overeat rarely helps us to change eating habits. We are so bogged down by the numerous "reasons" we dig up that we end up feeling more confused than ever. A necessary step in the right direction is learning how to acknowledge the influence of the past without letting it dominate your present or your future.

In our society, we're hooked on the idea of understanding "why." Why do I overeat when I know I'll feel lousy tomorrow? Why can't I control myself and eat only half of the bag of chips? Why can't I resist the smell of fresh-baked bread? Knowing your history of behavior is important, but coming up with a plan that gets you moving in the direction of change is the only understanding that will ultimately make a difference.

Let yesterday go, for if you don't it will hang around your neck like a dead albatross and drag you down."
- **Leo Buscaglia**

3. Lower Your Expectations

There must be more to life than having everything!
- Maurice Sendak

When you imagine your "ideal self," do you envision cavorting around the beach in a skimpy bikini, as slender and willowy as one of the models in a magazine? At least it's a positive goal, you might think. However, contrary to current notions of "common sense," this *positive* way of thinking may actually hinder your ability to maintain a reasonable weight.

In his book *The Paradox of Choice: Why More is Less*, author Barry Schwartz analyzes a wide range of research findings and presents some unusual advice for reaching our goals. The following "uncommon-sense" lessons may be particularly relevant for those of us who struggle with the issue of recurring weight gain.

- We would be better off if we lowered our expectations
- We would be better off seeking the "good enough" instead of "the best"

Such findings appear to fly in the face of conventional wisdom. Shouldn't we set high expectations? Shouldn't we "think big"? Yet, if it were that easy, we'd all be rich, skinny, and very, very satisfied.

Mr. Schwartz doesn't argue that more choice and high expectations are bad—only that aiming too high can bring about the opposite of what we are hoping for. Though most of us know what it's like to set a firm goal only to throw in the towel a short time later, our culture tells us that "aiming for less" is hardly a worthwhile endeavor.

WOULD YOU RATHER FEEL SATISFIED WITH "GOOD ENOUGH" OR MAKE YOURSELF MISERABLE SEEKING THE ULTIMATE?

Back in the days when I was struggling with my weight, I came across an exercise program that made the claim that following their routine on a regular basis could make a person's legs appear longer. Apparently the exercise would stretch the muscles. Thrilled by the idea that my short legs could actually appear lean and long, I purchased the video and hurried home, eager to get started. But alas, after watching the tall, thin women as they went through round after round of boring repetitions, I became so discouraged that by the time I finished watching the video, I'd also munched my way through a whole bag of cookies. The only lesson I took away from the experience was the futility of trying. No matter how much effort I put in, I was never going to look like those models.

The exercise routine would have been beneficial if I'd stuck with it and, with leaner muscles, my legs might have appeared a bit longer. So why did yet another perfectly good idea end up with me eating cookies instead of exercising? The problem is that, similar to "one-size-fits-all" pantyhose, many programs designed to fit everyone simply don't fit the individual.

> *The shoe that fits one person pinches another;*
> *there is no recipe for living that suits all cases.*
> **- Carl Jung**

No matter how great a diet plan or exercise method might seem, you need to take into account the way your emotional side will respond. If it gets spooked, you'll probably end up like me, munching on snacks and trying *not* to think about yet another failure.

To this day, I don't do rigorous exercise but instead try to incorporate activity into my daily life because I've never been motivated enough to follow a strict, demanding exercise routine. Call me lazy, or maybe I just don't care enough. Either way, I learned that I had to formulate a plan that uniquely suited me or I wouldn't stick with it.

Your rational side can come up with a long list of excellent reasons for doing something, but if the plan doesn't engage your powerful emotional side, you won't get far. You'll just get stuck with an unruly elephant on your hands.

I have learned that seeking "good enough" instead of constantly struggling within the yo-yo diet trap works so much better for me. At the same time, I am well aware that there is plenty of room for improvement. Therefore, I continue to pick-and-choose as I work toward adding better habits to my day-to-day life.

- Can you think of times when you have set a commendable goal only to give up before achieving what you set out for?
- What do you do differently when you reach a goal?
- Can you think of a time when your weight was "good enough" yet you were still dissatisfied?
- Do you ever make yourself miserable by raising the bar too high and setting yourself up for failure?

Seeking "good enough" is an effective way of decreasing your failure rate. However, as the next uncommon sense concept explains, dealing with feelings of failure is one of those facts of life that cannot always be avoided.

4. Prepare For Failure

Life is under no obligation to give us what we expect.
-                - Margaret Mitchell

An insidious sense of failure is one of those self-destructive feelings that can undermine our good efforts. As a result, when we encounter a setback, we may feel convinced that our best attempts have proven futile and there's no hope. It's easy to forget that failure is a part of life and learning—and so is getting up and moving on.

> Gloria has been struggling to keep her weight stable after losing several pounds. Her fear is that she'll lose control and backslide into an eating binge, so she tries to keep strict watch over her food consumption each and every day. She's been managing quite well until recently, when she agreed to meet some friends for a social evening. She started the evening firm in her decision to have a light salad and only one glass of wine. But as the table filled with cheese-covered nachos and mouth-watering chicken wings, she gave in and ate more than she intended.
> On the way home, Gloria experienced an overwhelming sense of gloom. "I'm always so weak," she lamented. "I'll never be able to control my eating habits. I've gone and blown all my good efforts." So what did she do next? Stop at the store and pick up a carton of ice cream that she proceeded to polish off as soon as she got home. To make matters worse, her belief that she had wiped out her hard work spiraled her back into an all-or-nothing pattern and she binged until she'd gained back her weight.

Researcher and author Martin Seligman, Ph.D., advocate of positive psychology, gives insight into Gloria's reaction in his book *Learned Optimism: How to Change Your Mind and Your Life*. Apparently, Gloria is suffering from a condition known as "Learned Helplessness," a thinking trap triggered by repeated failure. As a result, she has come to believe that her attempts to change will always be unsuccessful. Thus she experiences a mindless sense of futility that clouds her ability to see how she's creating a mountain out of a minor obstacle.

Consider for a moment how you think about the causes of your misfortunes. According to Seligman, if a setback makes you think, "It's me, it's going to last forever, it's going to undermine everything I do," then your explanatory style is likely undermining your efforts to make a change.

If that's the case, then why don't you just stop those thoughts? Well, it's a bit more complicated than that. Most of us don't understand the process that creates our emotions. We think of a feeling as...well...a feeling, without recognizing the close affinity between thoughts, feelings and the words we say to ourselves. Yet the best way to reduce a self-destructive feeling is to catch the negative self-talk that it's attached to before it translates into a negative behavior. As much as a feeling can seem overwhelming, the behavior is what counts in the end.

> **Words differently arranged have a different meaning and meanings differently arranged have a different effect.**
>
> **- Blaise Pascal**

For example, when Gloria ate too many chicken wings and nachos, if she had just snared those first pessimistic words and countered her own negative explanations, she might have said, "Hold on a minute. So maybe I did eat more than I intended, but I've been doing pretty well over-all. I'll have a good sleep tonight and eat lean and healthy tomorrow."

- Can you relate to Gloria's thinking trap?
- How would you advise Gloria to "talk back" to her pessimistic thoughts?

5. Expect Fear

To fear is one thing. To let fear grab you by the tail and swing you around is another.
- Katherine Paterson

Say that you go for your yearly checkup and you're informed that, for the sake of your **FACE YOUR HIDDEN FEARS** health, you must lose twenty pounds and exercise at least forty minutes a day. The doctor hands you a sheet of paper listing the types of foods you should eat and those you need to avoid, then adds that you're in luck! You can join a weight management clinic and get measured and weighed every two weeks free of charge. All you have to do is agree to eat the right foods and exercise every day.

So, how lucky do you feel? Does your heart leap with joy at this fortunate opportunity to help you get in shape? If not, if you're assailed by a wild desire to rush out and buy your favorite comfort food, then you've been ambushed by—of all things—fear. You're not likely to recognize the feeling as fear, but it is. What's happening is that your amygdala, your primitive fight-or-flight response, is sending out red alert signals. Our minds were designed for survival back in ancient times when the amygdala's alert could have been signaling a lion hiding behind the next tree.

Today, we still need our fight-or-flight response for true moments of danger, such as hitting an icy patch on a road. In such cases it would make no sense to sit back and ponder what to do. Most of the time, however, that pesky amygdala is overreacting and interfering with the rational and creative side of your brain. Options shut down and all you see is the bad news: Exercise every day and give up my favorite foods. *No thanks*.

As irrational as this type of fear may be, the biggest mistake is to underestimate it. Remember, you can't control your emotional fear center—your inner-elephant—through sheer force. You need a strategy. You need to find a way to manage your emotions so you can bypass the fear and make the changes you desire.

- Are you aware of an uneasy feeling when you are faced with a choice that threatens your comfort zone?
- Do you recognize the feeling as "fear"?

The following section will show you the details of how to begin your own journey and how to go about it creatively, without arousing your emotional fear center. Are you ready to set yourself up for success instead of failure?

CHAPTER 3

THE POWER OF SMALL

*"A journey of a thousand miles must
begin with the first step."*

- Lao Tzu

.

Contemplating a change creates anxiety. Even a good change stirs up some trepidation. As a result, procrastination has a way of creeping in, just as it does before taking the plunge into a diet. Therefore, the next plan of action is to make use of a strategy that will enable you to take the first step without allowing procrastination to hamper your progress.

In The "Now"

Where are you now in terms of your goals? The only way to take a meaningful measurement of this is to keep a realistic outlook and respect your true self.

If, in the past, you had a tendency to reach your goal only to slide back once you were there, then it's important to do something different. Otherwise, you'll get more of the same.

Too often we think of weight in terms of success or failure. *"I'm overweight so I've failed at keeping myself thin."* Or, *"I've finally lost enough weight, so I've succeeded."* Unfortunately, if you gain back the weight, your self-esteem can take a sharp nosedive. Because self-esteem is wrapped up with our achievements—and idyllic success doesn't always last—we are at the mercy of a measuring stick imposed from the outside.

Only when you learn to measure yourself by your own standards will you feel at peace with who you are. There is no right answer to the question of how to attain your goals. What matters is that you respect all aspects of yourself, including your strengths, your limitations, and ultimately, your choices.

Knowing your starting point—*where you are now*—will not only help you to ground yourself in the present, but also to realistically consider where you need to be to satisfy yourself on your own terms. Keep the following two crucial points in mind as you begin:

- Ground yourself in the present—where you are now
- Do not judge where you are—be realistic

Following is a 10-Point Scale, a technique often used in Solution-Oriented Therapy. The 10-Point Scale can help you visualize both where you are now and the direction you are heading .

On a scale of 1 to 10, where are you currently in terms of your personal satisfaction with your weight?

SATISFACTION SCALE

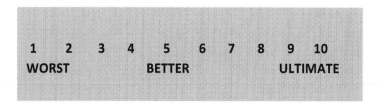

Go easy on yourself, and remember—no comparisons—measure yourself "on your own terms". Now take a good look in the mirror—smile—and realistically decide where you need to be in order to feel better about yourself. Not everybody can make a leap to the "ultimate" but everybody can feel "better."

> *"It is the greatest of all mistakes to do nothing because you can only do a little. Do what you can.*
> – Sidney Smith

My Small Treadmill Step

As you've probably deduced, I'm particularly resistant to organized, routine exercise. I try, but I must admit my drop-out rate has consistently been close to one hundred percent. Nevertheless, I did find a way to experience some success over the years. During one particularly cold, snowy winter, when I wasn't able to get away to warmer climates as I often do, I found myself feeling shut-in. My main activity is usually brisk walking, outside, so after several days of inactivity I decided to try out the treadmill in the condo activity room.

I didn't like treadmills and, as expected, the routine was so boring I almost quit. Nevertheless, I decided to set a small goal of ten minutes a day—at least a bit of movement. Surely I could handle ten minutes of boredom.

Ten minutes might hardly seem worth the effort, but once I got started, most days I wound up walking between thirty and forty minutes. Over time, my speed increased, and as I listened to music, I even came to enjoy the process. Yet I often felt resistance as the time for my walk approached. So I'd tell myself "just ten minutes" and my resistance would melt away. Every once in a while I did walk only ten minutes, but even that made me feel good—knowing that I hadn't let my *irrational resistance* get the better of me.

This might not seem like a big accomplishment, but for me it was an important step. After a few weeks, I started to notice that I could run up the stairs with ease and I felt stronger and more alert. The benefits put me in a more receptive state of mind when I considered other modes of exercise

The key point of this example is that I found a strategy to get past my resistance. By simply lowering the bar on my expectations, I was able to tiptoe around my fear and just go ahead and do it. This is exactly what Robert Maurer, professor of behavioral sciences at UCLA, suggests in his brilliant book *One Small Step Can Change Your Life–The Kaizen Way*.

Dr. Maurer describes Kaizen as "a natural, graceful technique for achieving goals and maintaining excellence." A tactic used by savvy Japanese businesses for decades as well as by private citizens throughout the world, it's a simple, small-step strategy that most of us already know yet don't truly appreciate. When I read Maurer's explanation, I recognized that in my own way, I have used similar small-step strategies as the basis for changing and managing my eating and activity habits over the years.

On the other hand, the typical North American way of making a change is what Maurer describes as "innovation"—the opposite of Kaizen. Innovation requires a "big leap" change. Diets are a good example of innovation. How many times have you seen a commercial advertising a revolutionary diet endorsed by a celebrity who has lost a large amount of weight in a short amount of time?

When it works, innovation is great. People feel pride and a sense of control. As we know, however, the vast majority of people who lose weight on a restrictive diet—no matter how revolutionary—gain it back. Even the rich and famous. The fact is, while innovation works in the short term, in the long term it often fails.

So if the radical method of big, quick change has backfired for you, then Kaizen offers a safe, no-fail alternative.

But here is the rule: *You have to aim for "small"*.

I'll EXERCISE 5 MINUTES A DAY FOR ONE WEEK THEN 6 MINUTES NEXT WEEK

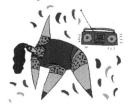

Slower Can Be Better

Crawling still gets you there.
- Cynthia Copeland-Lewis

As noted previously, fear of change is rooted in your brain's physiology; therefore, when your fight-or-flight response is aroused, you experience an uncomfortable emotion—call it stress, anxiety, or fear. This happens not only when you are facing a crisis, but also when you're faced with something as seemingly minor as giving up a favorite food. Just thinking about self-denial is often enough to raise your stress level and shut down the rational, creative side of your brain. Next thing you know, you're heading for the comfort of a favorite snack.

The small-step method allows you to sidestep the fear and come up with tiny, creative ways to outwit your emotional fear center. But how small is small?

Robert Maurer describes this point most eloquently in his book when he relates the story of Julie, a young woman referred to the clinic where he worked.

A single mother with soaring stress, excess weight and high blood pressure, she was a candidate for depression, heart disease and stroke. The resident talked to her about the need to make changes for the sake of her health and was about to prescribe the usual thirty minutes a day of aerobic exercise when Dr. Maurer spoke up: "How about if you just march in front of the television, each day, for one minute?" Julie brightened and quickly agreed, and when she returned the following week she happily reported her success.

Of course, one minute a day was not going to make a differ-
ence in the long run, but at least she didn't drop out of the
program, which she'd done before. She even asked what else
she could do in one minute a day. Thus started her progress,
and over a period of time Julie incorporated enough exercise
and other healthy changes into her daily routine to make a
difference in her health.

Another reason the small-step strategy is so powerful is that it takes very little time. You can incorporate a small, easy change into your daily routine, and, with nothing to fear and no reason to stop, your brain has plenty of time to create new nerve pathways. Time-limited diets, on the other

BAD HABITS GAIN STRENGTH OVER TIME... BUT SO DO GOOD ONES!

hand, do not last long enough for your brain to build this new "software." And what does the new software do? It enables you to create new habits. Just as bad habits gradually gain strength over time, so do good ones.

Make Use of Small Rewards

**One of the secrets in life is to make stepping-stones
out of stumbling blocks.**
- Jack Penn

Small steps allow you to set your mental compass without creating the resistance that commonly happens when you aggressively push yourself into a big leap of change. But there is another component that helps to give that extra boost. And that is the power of small rewards.

As human beings, we want to feel good about our achievements, but if we only value big payoffs then we overlook the power of small, incremental changes. Yet one of the main reasons that people feel unmotivated in many areas of their lives is because they feel "underappreciated". Just think of how many small achievements you fail to notice. For example, if you walk for five minutes on the treadmill are you likely to feel good about your effort? Or are you more apt to say, "I'm so lazy. I only walked for five minutes."

Remember that you don't have to wait for someone else to encourage you or praise your efforts. Learn to focus on the small, genuine efforts that you make. Become conscious of those efforts and praise yourself—then you'll be more likely to repeat them.

Large rewards can become a goal in and of themselves. Small rewards are intrinsically satisfying because they boost your spirits and make you feel better. However, make sure that the reward is appropriate to the goal. For weight related goals it's best to stick with small rewards, such as a relaxing bubble-bath, or a small inexpensive gift. And make good use of praise. Instead of focusing on how little you did, focus on how great it is that you did a "little" better.

- What is one tiny step that you can take today to cut a few calories?
- How will you reward yourself for the small, yet worthy, achievement?

A man cannot be comfortable without his own approval.

\- **Mark Twain**

CHAPTER 4

ILLUMINATE YOUR
JOURNEY GOAL

If you aim at nothing, you'll hit it every time.
– Zig Ziglar

W hen you think of a journey, do you envision yourself wandering around aimlessly? Or do you have
a destination—a goal? Most plans begin with a goal as a
motivating factor, yet the process can vary greatly. Your
goal might be to reach your destination as quickly as possible, such as a diet. Or it might be to explore and learn in a
way that creates a lasting change. Whether a quick destination or a process, your will measure your success by whether
or not you attain your goal.

The Success Secret

Researchers Chip and Dan Heath, authors of *Switch: How to Change When Change is Hard*, highlight two significant, yet seemingly trivial, factors that often get in the way of successful goal attainment.

First, they discovered that when a goal is vague and lacks clear direction, our rational side is far more likely to get sidetracked. For example, a decision to "eat healthy and lose weight" is a good idea, but what exactly does that mean? Healthy eating is a fuzzy concept until you have a precise plan of action. As a result, when an attempt to make a change doesn't work, you might conclude that you are resistant to what's good for you. But the research points to a different possibility: Your resistance might be due to a simple lack of clarity.

Second, the researchers found that even when a goal is motivated by fearful statistics that convince our rational side of the need for change, most of us manage to ignore the facts. For example, knowing that saturated fat raises your statistical odds of heart disease, diabetes and other serious health problems, doesn't move your emotions anywhere near as much as the crackling sound when you open a bag of Cheez Doodles.

Over time, your rational side gets tired of trying to convince your emotional side to choose an apple or yogurt instead. What happens then? Most people give in to the high calorie snack. So here's the second possibility that research reveals: You might think you're just too lazy to keep on the right path, when really, your rational side is exhausted. Not only does this information put a different spin on why some goals are so difficult to reach, but it also gives us two more tools to help construct a successful change process.

Not only does this information put a different spin on why some goals are so difficult to reach, but it also gives us two more tools to help construct a successful change process. Instead of exhausting your rational side with futile attempts to coax your emotions into line, you can use these psychological tools to chisel out a path that will be easier to follow:

1. A motivation that will inspire the emotions
2. A step-by-step script, much like a recipe

Interestingly, both of these elements are contained in the very thing we want to avoid: A diet. We also know the main reason people keep going back to diets is because they work. So let's take a little side trip and explore the precise ingredients that make a diet work. After all, you're now in the business of gathering clues, creating a personal roadmap, and opening the door to possibilities.

Decipher A Diet

Why do diets work? Some diets promise that they can make you lose weight in record time while others guarantee you will lose weight in all the right places. Still others claim that a specific combination of foods will "melt away fat." In spite of so many competing claims, the plain truth is embarrassingly simple: If you follow the instructions, just about any diet will work.

But pay attention to the "if". For even if a diet claims to have mysterious qualities, you still have to follow the instructions. Therein lies the paradox. If you don't follow the formula with a fair amount of precision, it won't work.

Keeping in mind what we have learned, let's explore how diets manage to incorporate the two above success strategies. First of all, how does a diet manage to inspire our resistant emotional side enough to accept the deprivation? Although imminent health issues motivate some people, we humans tend to be moved to action by more shallow desires such as wanting to fit into an outfit for a specific event, or to trim down before a summer vacation. Appearance is still the No. 1 inspiration when it comes to dieting. Who would have thought our inner-con would be so susceptible to vanity?

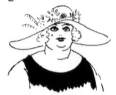

I WONDER IF I'LL FIT INTO MY LITTLE PINK DRESS IF I GO ON THE FAT-MELTING DIET?

Now let's examine the second success component. You're inspired enough to take the plunge—to really lose some weight. So how do you go about it? Do you make a vague plan such as, "I'll cut out junk food and eat more vegetables?" Or do you choose a specific diet with precise and clear instructions?

Most of us go for the clear-cut directions that a diet provides—in other words, a step-by-step script. If you follow it as you would a formula, you will have a prescription for success. With clear instructions in hand, you're far less likely to go wandering down the cookie aisle to check out whether those chocolate puffs might be on sale. Instead, you head straight for the sections that contain the foods on your diet.

The Fatal Flaw

Diets clearly contain two of the most important elements necessary to create a successful plan. They begin with an inspiring motivation that engages your emotions. And, no matter which diet you choose, it will provide a clear script. But there is a third factor that makes us tolerate the restrictions of a diet. Diets are time-limited. You're not making a commitment to live on cabbage soup and bananas for the rest of your life. *And therein lies the fatal flaw inherent in diets.* A diet only works as long as you follow the script with precision. Once you stop, if you are like most people, you will gain back the weight. Eventually, both your body and your self-esteem pay the price of the yo-yo diet syndrome.

Diets Are Time limited – Weight Is NOT

Understanding why and how diets work can help you to shape a formula for success in constructing your weight-loss strategy. Use the best of what diets have to offer, but discard the rest.

Remember:
- You need to motivate your emotional side
- You need a step-by-step recipe for success
- But...you don't want a rigid, time-limited formula

Your next step is to create an itinerary that includes the above elements, yet doesn't scare the elephant or exhaust the trainer. Because the journey is going to last a lot longer than two weeks, the challenge is to work out a strategy that will satisfy both your rational and your emotional sides at the same time.

Your First Small Step

Remember, you're embarking on one of those delicious, long, meandering journeys where you relax and soak up the atmosphere and information; where you are out of your usual comfort zone and therefore in the mood to take in uncommon information and try different things. As part of the leisurely pace, you have several small destination points to explore. Who doesn't like that kind of journey? Even your resistant emotional side could get excited about that.

Now take a minute and look back at the 10-point scale and revisit where you placed yourself. Say, for example, you put yourself at a four. Looking forward, where do you want to be? Keep in mind that the object of your goal is to feel "good enough" about yourself while also allowing you to enjoy food.

Perhaps you can think of a time when you were dissatisfied with your weight and now, in retrospect, you would be happy if you could be that weight again. Well life is often like that when we keep setting unrealistic goals; we miss the simple pleasure of "now". We diminish our reserve of "wellbeing" when we live life as if we're trying to win a beauty contest or win a race to reach a final outcome.

Okay, now back to the 10-point scale. Say you chose seven as your destination. That's still three points to cover, and depending on how you personally measure yourself, this could represent anywhere from a few pounds to maybe twenty or more pounds. Just thinking about the changes it will take to reach that goal can be enough to spook anybody's emotional side. Therefore, your strategy needs to be gentle enough so that you don't create resistance within yourself.

The sure way to achieve this is to come up with a first, small step. Remember "Julie" in Dr. Maurer's example? She started by marching in front of the TV for only one minute a day. Similarly, you want to choose an action that you can do most days without any major interruption to your lifestyle.

The beauty of this small step approach is that you eliminate the need to psych yourself up for a big change. No preparation and no pig-out before starting a diet next Monday. Your goal is to set yourself up for success—to move in the direction of "better" rather than a quick weight loss that only gives temporary satisfaction.

> ### TO A GREAT MIND NOTHING IS LITTLE
> ### - SHERLOCK HOLMES

On the other hand, it's important that this change be something you can actually do most days and fits in with your daily routine. Time and repetition are what habits are made of, and the easier and more mindless the change, the better your brain will accept the new behavior.

That's where the crystal-clear script comes in. Instead of making a decision to just cut back on pasta or eat more vegetables and fewer snacks, you need a measurable change that you can consciously integrate into your day-to-day routine. In fact you are probably already doing several small things randomly that would make a difference if you incorporated them into your daily life.

For example, do you sometimes choose a less calorie laden snack for a coffee break? Do you sometimes forego sugar or take less in your tea or coffee? Until you recognize the significance of small changes, you won't notice them. Once you do, however, you can make a conscious decision to amplify the change and make it work for you. So watch for clues in your everyday life and you will soon catch yourself doing something right!

Looking back on my personal experiences, I recall a particular incident of serendipity that fits the recipe for a small, successful change. Just as with my previous accidental change that was sparked by trying on my jeans, I didn't recognize the significance of this one at first. But by this time I was more alert to the importance of small changes.

> **FOOD FOR THOUGHT!**
>
> *100 calories a day add up to 5 lbs. in six months.*
>
> *Six months from now— would you rather lose or gain 5 lbs.?*

This episode occurred during a time in my life when my main mode of transportation was the bus. I was on my way home after work, feeling tired and somewhat weary. Gazing out the window, absentmindedly watching the buildings slide by, for some unknown reason I thought of my grandmother and how whenever she felt worn out, she'd make a cup of tea.

The thought appealed, and when I got home I went and put on the kettle. Although my usual habit was to have a slice of toast and jam before dinner, that day I just had tea. I put up my feet and slowly sipped the warm drink while planning dinner and the evening ahead.

That was it. A small departure from my normal routine. I didn't give it any more thought until the next day at the same time, when I automatically went to prepare my toast. Then I remembered the tea and how refreshing it had been. I put on the kettle and sat back and enjoyed the age-old comfort of sipping the hot beverage. As I did so, a thought occurred to me. Why not make a cup of tea my pre-dinner habit instead of toast and jam?

And that's what I did. What's more, the tea habit became such a pleasant part of my routine that I bought a special cup to enhance the process. Simple and seemingly trivial, but it was one of those steps that made a difference in more ways than one.

> *The art of the tea way consists simply of boiling water, preparing tea and drinking it.*
> *- Rikyu*

Now, after reading the research, I realize why that small step was so easy to make into a habit. It contains the exact ingredients that make a plan more likely to work.

Motivation: On my way home I anticipated the calming process of making and drinking the tea—a simple motivation that soothed my emotions.

A Clear Script: When I walked in the door my rational side was in charge and knew the exact steps to take. I put on the kettle, first thing. Then prepared the tea, sat back and let the warm beverage ease my weariness away.

Nothing vague or difficult about that. The tea replaced my old habit of toast and jam, yet didn't leave me feeling deprived. As a result, over time my brain made new software and formed a new habit—one that saved me at least 100 calories a day!

You can begin to build success by creating a simple script for one, tiny change. It will only take a few minutes:

- List several small, food choice changes that you could do that don't feel like a big deal
- Rather than thinking in terms of "changing" a habit, think more of "tweaking" a behavior as a way to *save and shave a few calories*
- Choose one small change that you can repeat daily
- Keep it up until you do it without thinking

Because our minds are so complex and our emotional sides carry so much weight, we must continue to raise our awareness, prepare for the inevitable setbacks, and stock up on more ways to keep the emotional side from gaining too much power.

The next section will introduce you to another psychological roadblock. So get ready to learn about "mindsets" and what you can do to guard yourself against this insidious thinking trap that can easily drag you off path if you don't recognize it for what it is.

CHAPTER 5

DON'T BELIEVE EVERYTHING YOU THINK

Every man, wherever he goes, is encompassed by a
cloud of comforting convictions, which move
with him like flies on a summer day.
- Bertrand Russell

To help us further understand the power of our thoughts, psychologist Carol Dweck uses the term "mindsets" to describe our divided mind. In more than twenty years of research, she has discovered that most people fall into one of two camps:

- fixed mindset non-learners
- growth mindset learners

Furthermore, she found that children as young as four already fit one of these two categories. Children with a fixed mindset believe kids who are born smart "don't do mistakes," and they were reluctant to try anything new.

By contrast, children with the growth mindset welcomed the challenge of learning new things—even if it meant making mistakes along the way. Originally, I assumed that the lucky ones who were talented and/or didn't have difficulty learning new things would automatically be growth minded "learners" whereas people like me—those who have to put more effort into learning—would naturally be more reluctant to test their abilities. Surprisingly, that's not true.

Dr. Dweck found that ability and intelligence have little effect on mindset. In fact, some of the brightest and most talented students avoided challenges and effort 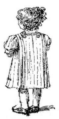 **I DON'T WANT A CHALLENGE. MY MIND IS FIXED.** while some of the less brilliant students thrived in the face of new, demanding tasks, succeeding through persistence.

So, what is the defining factor that makes some people more growth-minded and some more fixed-minded? And, if we are stuck in a fixed-mindset, can we change?

The first message for those who struggle with food habits is that intelligence has nothing to do with body weight. Education and talent do not automatically bestow better self-control or make it easier for you to maintain a satisfactory weight. Don't let anyone tell you that weight is a measure of your brain power.

Secondly, Professor Dweck tells us that fixed mindset people can learn to identify this tendency and incorporate strategies of a growth mindset into their lives at any point.

Your Learning Style

Here's a short quiz to help you recognize your mindset when it comes to weight management. Decide which of the following statements apply to you and which do not:

1. When I diet I am motivated by a desire to prove that I can succeed.

2. I welcome effort even though it requires a bit of a learning curve.

3. When I encounter a setback I feel embarrassed by a sense of failure.

4. Mistakes are good because they help me learn something new.

5. Deep down I believe that people who aren't overweight are just "lucky" and don't have to work at it.

6. I see failure as an opportunity for future growth.

7. I believe that if a person is smart or lucky they shouldn't have to exert effort to succeed.

8. I think that effort is more praiseworthy than talent or ability.

9. I tend to keep repeating something I believe, in the hope that it will work next time.

10. I am more likely to try something new rather than repeat what hasn't worked in the past.

If you answered "yes" to 2, 4, 6, 8 and 10, you already lean toward a growth mindset. "Yes" to the odd numbers means you need some work to build up your growth mindset.

Just as we did with Seligman's categories of explanatory style, it's important to identify our mindset as a tool to raise awareness. If you recognize that you tend toward a fixed mindset, you can take the steps to become "growth" minded instead, and then make good use of the benefits to help change your relationship with food. Remember, the defining difference between fixed and growth minded people is their openness to the idea of a challenge. So when you are faced with a challenge, remind yourself that a little effort can lead to a big spurt in growth

Update Your Mindset

My strength lies solely in my tenacity.
– Louis Pasteur

Back when I saw the first glimmer of hope that there might be other options to the way I had always approached eating and diets, I still resisted putting any effort into figuring out how it had happened. After all, my amygdala was sending out fear signals, reminding me that I didn't want to get hooked back into my obsession with weight. I'd pretty much convinced myself that I only had two alternatives: either stringent dieting or gaining weight. No wonder my emotions had me locked in fear mode. With my brain stuck in a "fixed mindset", I'd cornered myself into an "either-or" way of thinking.

However, once I allowed even the slender prospect of another possibility to enter my brain, I began to notice other aspects of my life that suggested unrecognized options might exist.

For example, I had long since accepted the "fact" that I simply didn't have what it takes to be an "achiever." Like many young people who didn't excel in any special way, I believed that we either have it or we don't (a common way of thinking in those days). The fact that I typically needed to put diligent effort into any achievement gave credence to my belief that, obviously, I didn't have what it takes.

Yet despite my lack of belief in myself, I had recently started a change process in another area of my life when I 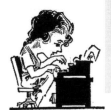 **I MAY NOT BE BRILLIANT BUT PERSISTENCE WINS IN THE END** had applied and been accepted to the university for admission as a mature student. My negative side still believed that I'd only passed the entrance exams by sheer luck and that before long "they"—whoever "they" are—would find out that I really didn't have what it takes and expel me from the program. Still, a little voice inside reminded me that I had passed the entrance exam. Which only proved—I thought—that even without talent, you can sometimes outwit fate.

Clearly I lacked self-confidence, but nevertheless the very idea that persistence—tenacity—had opened the door to a new possibility in one area of my life gave me hope that it might pay off in another. With a little determination, maybe I could discover what to do differently to maintain an acceptable weight. So I watched and waited and before long, my first bit of evidence was revealed.

A Clue

My first concrete clue came the weekend after I discovered my non-diet weight loss. I'd baked a cake, as was my pattern each Sunday. After dinner I settled down to have dessert while watching Walt Disney with my young son. I was thinking how wonderful the cake and ice cream tasted, when it suddenly occurred to me that I hadn't had dessert since the Sunday before. I'd been busy every evening doing homework since I started the university term and hadn't had time to indulge in my usual evening activity of snacking in front of the TV.

Immediately, I got out my little notebook—detectives need notebooks—and wrote down my first bit of evidence.

> **IT IS, OF COURSE, A TRIFLE, BUT THERE IS NOTHING SO IMPORTANT AS TRIFLES.**
> **– SHERLOCK HOLMES**

Have cut down on television and snacking since starting classes. But then I remembered that homework was only a temporary situation; once the holidays came I'd automatically go back to my usual routine. Unless I made a calculated plan that I could stick to. So in my notebook I wrote: *"No snacking with TV during the week. Dessert only on Sunday."*

I realized my plan wouldn't always be easy. I'd have to learn to improvise. Yet the evidence was clear—I'd found one small change that worked. I could probably find more. I looked down at the cake and ice cream on my plate and an old saying popped into my mind: "You can't have your cake and eat it too."

Well, *maybe they were wrong.* I was having my cake, and I was pretty sure if I kept to my once-a-week dessert plan, I would soon fit into my jeans, too.

- Can you think of a time when persistence, instead of talent, paid off and you attained success in something you wanted?
- Do you sometimes doubt your own "self-doubt" because deep down you know that a small effort is really what makes the difference?

CHAPTER 6

YOUR BUILT-IN COMPUTER

Knowledge is learning something every day.
Wisdom is letting go of something every day.
                              - Zen Proverb

Have you ever experienced the heartbreak of having your computer crash, only to realize you haven't backed up some important information? Suddenly efficiency drops to floor level while all your mental and emotional energy is consumed by the frantic effort to replace whatever you can. Yesterday you could take the information for granted. Today it may feel as if you've lost an arm.

Your brain is like that, a computer holding an infinite amount of information, a collective data bank of details you have retained over a lifetime. You want a cup of coffee? The thought has only to flash into your mind before the information is at your fingertips and you're filling the coffee maker.

Too easy, you say? Just try getting a new machine with all sorts of extra knobs and dials. Suddenly the task isn't so simple. Once we learn something, be it simple or complex, good or bad, the process of accomplishing the task becomes mindless.

Clearly, if we had to live without our "mindless" database, our level of efficiency would plummet. After all, how many of us could find our way to work if we couldn't find our way around a coffee maker?

The ability to function mindlessly is an essential part of efficient living. If our cosmic database suddenly crashed like a computer's, we'd lose a good part of our survival skills.

IS "JUNK MAIL" OVERWHELMING THE GOOD INFORMATION IN YOUR MINDLESS DATA BASE?

Yet, over time, we also collect a lot of useless "junk mail," which unfortunately has a way of sticking just as securely as the useful data. Our brains are so resourceful at taking in the information we feed it that we often learn a process without realizing how firmly it's sticking. But once that information sticks—you have created a habit.

Fortunately, most of our habits are beneficial and even necessary for our survival. Nevertheless, as proficient as our cosmic database may be at responding to cues and retrieving good information, it's equally quick to retrieve the bad. And the majority of us have collected at least a few bad habits along the way, ready to be triggered by the smallest cue. Furthermore, when we want to get rid of a bad habit, we can't just hit "delete." Unlike a computer, we don't come equipped with a "trash" center that we can empty with the click of a mouse.

The line between "mindful" and "mindless" is indeed fine. As part of the quest to achieve a more "mindful" state and raise awareness, we need to understand how "trash" ends up in our mindless zone and how to become more efficient at filing good habits instead of bad into our cosmic database.

How We Make Mindless Habits

According to food psychologists, we make as many as 200 food-related choices a day. We'd be nervous wrecks if we deliberated each and every one. We learn to choose efficiently without expending energy on each routine decision such as what kind of cereal to buy and whether to have our coffee black or with cream. But what happens when you're suddenly confronted with a new choice?

Say you're having coffee with a friend. She orders the Frappuccino, telling you that it's scrumptious and you must try one. You ponder. Should you? It does look awfully good and your regular coffee seems dull by comparison. But it's more expensive and probably fattening.

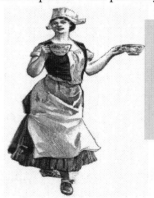

WILL THAT BE COFFEE
WITH CREAM FOR 50
CALORIES?
OR FRAPPUCCINO FOR
250 CALORIES?

Today the decision is *not* mindless. You struggle a bit with the choice. But say you order the new coffee and love it. Even though you don't intend to make it a habit, you end up having the Frappuccino for the next two weeks. Although you did not make a conscious decision to create a new habit, after a couple of weeks you barely give it a thought. The coffee shop has become the prompt that sends the question to your cosmic database, and when the waiter asks for your order your reply is mindless, without hesitation: "A Frappuccino, please." No wasted time or energy spent on trying to decide—you've now become a steady Frappuccino drinker and the decision is automatic. In other words, you've made a habit.

That's how small, seemingly irrelevant decisions end up in our vast mindless zone where choices and decisions are carried out on autopilot. With the hundreds of decisions we make in a day, you can see why we need quick, habitual responses to keep us sane. But six months later, you notice that your clothes seem to be getting a tad tight. Then you step on the scale and find that you've gained four pounds. What happened, you wonder. Do you immediately think of the Frappuccino?

> **FOOD FOR THOUGHT!**
> *A Frappuccino is 250 calorie or more. That can add up to 5 lbs. in 6 months!*

Not likely. After all, you don't gain several pounds from one Frappuccino or even a week of specialty coffees. But over several months, your body registers the increase in calories. Gradually a few pounds are added until you notice the difference all at once. But because of the time lapse and all of the other things going on in your life, you are likely to blame the weight gain on something unrelated, such as lack of exercise or getting older, while the real culprit goes unnoticed.

Changing and reshaping habits begins with an understanding of how to make use of our vast mindless zone, located in our cosmic database. It is this database that holds the key to managing our weight efficiently and with a minimum of pain and effort. Changing mindless habits is just one in a series of steps that take advantage of this database as a weight-loss tool.

How Mindless Habits Can Work for You

"I call intuition cosmic fishing. You feel the nibble and then you have to hook the fish."
– Buckminster Fuller

Unless you spend the rest of your life weighing and measuring everything you eat, you will, as a rule, consume close to the same amount of food each day within two to three hundred calories. This happens because of instinct and habit. We size up the amount on our plate, we tend to eat the same types of foods, and when we finish the amount we are used to, we know we've had enough. Somehow, we regulate our food intake each day so that it's fairly consistent.

Say you tend to eat about 2000 calories a day but today you're constantly on the run and only have time for a quick muffin. You notice the difference in calorie intake because you feel weak and cranky. Or there's a luncheon at an all-you-can-eat buffet and you overeat and end up consuming 1,000 calories more than usual. Your body notices and you groan and feel uncomfortable. The fact is, we are keenly aware when we eat significantly more or less than usual. However, according to Ph.D. Brian Wansink, author of *Mindless Eating: Why We Eat More Than We Think*, there is a margin of a couple hundred calories, more or less, which we don't notice.

That's why something like changing from a daily coffee with cream and one sugar to a Frappuccino coffee can go unnoticed. The difference will be anywhere from 100 to 300 calories, depending on whether you get the low fat or the higher fat variety. But in your mind it falls under the category of coffee, and if you choose the low-fat type you might even believe that there is no real difference in calorie content at all. Your body doesn't signal any discomfort from the extra calories, so the only information filed away is how good it tastes. Then next time you have another, and then another the next time, and so on until, unwittingly, you have formed a new habit that adds at least 100 calories to your daily consumption.

If all other variables remain the same, that small increase in calories—perhaps 150 extra per day—could add up to as much as twelve pounds in a year. That's twelve extra pounds—and you likely wouldn't even know where it came from. You can blame those extra, mysterious pounds on the middle-ground—the 200 calories, more or less—that your body and mind doesn't consciously register.

You don't notice a couple hundred calories more because that's not enough to make you feel stuffed. A stomach doesn't keep track of the number of calories or how many pretzels are eaten out of a large bag. On the other hand, you won't feel deprived if you eat a couple hundred calories fewer. It's basically an internal balancing act that keeps your weight stable.

This little fact, however, can be enormously useful to help you lose weight over a period of time because it eliminates the main reason that diets backfire. The "deprivation" problem. Eating 200 calories less will hardly register in your brain, which means you won't feel deprived.

Stuffed	Unconscious Border	Deprived
1000 more	200 more or less	1000 less

This "unconscious border" as noted above, is an excellent tool that you can consciously put to use. Instead of mindlessly gaining several pounds you can make a few small adjustments to your eating patterns and lose a few instead. Here are a couple of suggestions to help you get started.

First of all, tune in to your body signals. When you're half way through a meal, put down your fork and focus on how you feel. Are you getting full? Still hungry? Are you aiming to eat everything on your plate? Or do you just want to feel full enough?

Now, reflect on your last meal. Thinking back, how could you have cut a few calories just by paying attention? Do you tend to use sauces, dressings, marinades and such?

These products can add many hidden calories without your body noticing the extra consumption. You can learn to cut calories by using a bit less or experimenting with lighter versions. Reading labels is not such a big deal because we tend to use the same sauces over and over. So once you gather the information and pay attention to the subtlety of the flavors, you'll discover that you can cut calories simply by using a bit less or choosing a lighter version.

Making tiny, routine changes is a great way to sneak in some better eating habits without feeling deprived. Yet still, there is the matter of just "doing it" and many people believe that they don't have the willpower to make even these small changes.

Therefore, the next section, based on psychological traps, will take you on an inside tour of the habit-willpower connection. And you just might recognize some of the traps as ones that you fall into—completely unaware.

CHAPTER 7

THE HABIT-WILLPOWER CONNECTION

Experience is that wonderful thing that enables you to recognize a mistake when you make it again...(and again and again)!
- Unknown

Have you ever felt as if willpower and self-control are virtues passed out at birth that somehow you missed? Those who struggle with weight control often feel judged when their willpower deserts them. Many feel that a lack of willpower is a public measure not only of their waistline, but their very moral fibre.

Dr. Kelly McGonigal teaches a course at Stanford University on the Science of Self Control. In her book *The Willpower Instinct: How Self-Control Works, Why it Matters, and What You Can Do About it*, she points out we humans struggle with various forms of temptation, procrastination, addiction and other such inclinations that are part of the human condition.

In spite of the universality of this type of struggle, society as a whole still tends to judge any display of poor self-control; the result being that we desperately try to hide what we think of as our "weaknesses and personal inadequacies".

However, researchers now understand that there is more to willpower than strong will. In fact, willpower has a strong biological component and, much like a muscle, can be strengthened or weakened by the choices you make. That means you can learn what depletes your willpower as well as what strengthens it. Adding more "will" to your willpower can increase your success rate in growing better habits and making changes to old ones that are hard to budge.

Let's begin by thinking of self-control in terms of your own history. If you catch yourself making statements such as, "What's the matter with me? I just don't have any self-control," stop right there. Remind yourself that you are likely depleting your willpower reservoir but you are unaware of the process. The good news is that as you become more enlightened you will recognize what depletes your willpower and how to build up your supply so that you're not running on empty.

Remember my Sherlock Holmes approach? Once again, it's time to dig out your notebook and become a detective in your own life.

How We Lose Willpower

I can resist everything except temptation.
– Oscar Wilde

For fifteen years, researcher Roy Baumeister has studied the mysteries of willpower. In study after study, he found that the longer people used their self-control, the more depleted it became. When he asked people to concentrate on a task, he found their concentration tended to fade if the task went on too long. But surprisingly, so did their ability to do other tasks, including some requiring physical strength.

In other words, actions that require willpower, whether controlling your temper, resisting a chocolate chip cookie, or forcing yourself to concentrate when you're tired, all tap the same source of strength. Most of us equate willpower with resisting obvious temptations—the bag of Oreos, the blueberry pie in the bakery window—but when we look at all the actions and feelings that weaken the willpower muscle, it becomes clear why we often seem to run out of steam.

ARE YOU DEPLETING YOUR SUPPLY OF WILLPOWER?

The variety of behaviors that require strength of will—whether forcing yourself to sit through a boring meeting, navigating through traffic, or impressing a new friend—all drain a portion of your willpower. And what about the seemingly irrelevant decisions that consume energy because of the sheer number of choices, from choosing between ten different types of dishwasher soap to twenty-one flavors of ice cream? With each decision that you ponder, no matter how trivial, you use some of your supply of willpower.

Although it's encouraging to know that moments of indulgence are not a true measure of our inadequacies, nevertheless the sheer number of actions and reactions that exhaust willpower can make the effort to change seem overwhelming. Nevertheless, when it comes to understanding this new look at self-control, knowledge is power. The better you understand the concept, the less likely you are to mindlessly scatter your willpower on behaviors that are in your power to control.

The Willpower Muscle

The willpower muscle is different from the physical muscles in your body. It's not in the arm that reaches out and lifts that chocolate bar to your mouth, nor in the legs that refuse to go for a brisk walk in spite of your promises to do so. But because willpower can be weakened or strengthened by our activities, Baumeister came to think of it as a "muscle" situated in the brain. Repeated obligations that require self-control use up our brain's energy and therefore exhaust our willpower muscle.

Basically, the physical side of our willpower supply is fueled when our body converts energy from food to glucose. When researchers tested people who were glucose deprived, they discovered over and over that low glucose means low self-control. Even small behaviors requiring self-control resulted in large drops in the brain's store of glucose.

Imagine this: You've just arrived home after one of those days. You're grumpy, stressed, and don't feel like cooking.

Nevertheless, you draw on your last bit of willpower and resolve to prepare a healthy, lean meal. Just then the phone rings and you're reminded that you made a commitment to go for a mile-long walk with a neighbor. You vaguely recall that when you made the commitment you envisioned yourself feeling energized by a walk followed by a healthy meal.

What had you been thinking? The very thought of exercise followed by cooking exhausts you, so you reach into the cupboard and take out your stash of chocolate chip cookies, digging in and devouring as many as you can to boost your energy for the exertion ahead.

Most of us know what it's like to reach for something sweet for a quick rush of energy. Once in awhile this method can be useful, but the quick-fix backfires when blood sugar spikes and then falls too rapidly, causing even greater hunger and intense cravings for sweets.

FOOD FOR THOUGHT:
- **Impulsive behavior is fueled by a low glucose supply to your brain**
- **A steady supply of glucose strengthens Willpower**
- **Sweets cause blood sugar to spike & crash**

This crash and burn effect can cause "willpower burnout," where you find yourself craving more of what you really don't want, yet feel less able to resist. In order to protect yourself against this type of burnout, it's important to recognize the common, yet tricky willpower traps that can snare you when you are least aware.

Willpower Traps

Habit is stronger than reason.
— **George Santayana**

Armed with some knowledge of the inner life of will-power, you should feel less inclined to blame yourself if you just don't have enough self-control. But how can you conserve your strength-of-will for when you really need it? It's not as if you can pull up to a "willpower pump" and fill up when you're running low. As with most learning experiences, the first step is to raise your awareness so that you can gain insight into some of the ways you may be squandering your willpower's energy.

The following Willpower Traps are some of the most common that unwittingly capture us. See if you recognize yourself as falling prey to any of them.

It is a capital mistake to theorize before you have all the evidence. It biases the judgment.
-Sherlock Holmes

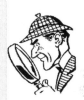

False Hope Trap

If you keep doing what you've been doing
you'll keep getting what you got...

University of Toronto psychologists Janet Polivy and Peter Herman have studied the baffling question of why people keep repeating efforts to change even after they continue to fail over time. Like the character in the movie Groundhog Day, when it comes to weight management, are we doomed to repeat the same failures over and over?

HAVE YOU TRIED THE HOT-DOG DIET, YET?

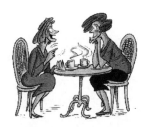

Polivy and Herman call this tendency to repeat the same mistakes the "false hope syndrome." This behavior is seen often enough in our society's inclination to believe that the next diet really will work regardless of past evidence.

Basically, we go through the same process over and over—following a restrictive diet, losing some weight, then inevitably gaining it back—ending up where we started, if not worse off.

Researchers acknowledge that our society promotes instant gratification, and many programs are marketed to encourage belief in unrealistic expectations. As a result, people are brainwashed into believing the next diet will be the magic cure that will melt away the fat with minimal expenditure of time and effort.

Dr. Polivy hopes that people will begin to see that most quick-fix solutions are misleading. She also notes that we should become aware of the insidious nature of such faddish programs and how blithely they offer ridiculous promises. What's more, there are few controls on the claims that can be made, so it's a matter of "buyer beware".

Does this mean it's impossible to find a balance between the human inclination to want to indulge and the equally powerful desire to maintain a trim figure? Wouldn't we be better off to just give up? Not at all. The same researchers also found that some people do attain success, even after repeated failures. The reason for their success seems to be a willingness to make changes instead of repeating the same routine. Once they realize their current strategy isn't working, these people learn from their mistakes and make adjustments. However, in order to do so, they have to let go of wishing for a quick solution and take a more realistic approach.

Moving from a fixed mindset toward a growth mindset can be difficult when everybody else is doing more of the same. Albert Einstein recognized this human inclination long ago when he so aptly stated, *"Insanity is doing the same thing over and over again and expecting different results."*

- Do you have a tendency to do more of the same, even when the strategy has not worked in the past?
- What stops you from trying something different?

"For Your Own Good" Trap

One evening I was out for dinner with a group of friends.

PLEASE DON'T TELL ME WHAT I ALREADY KNOW

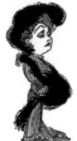

At the end of the meal, a waiter wheeled a cart laden with cakes and pastries to our tableside. The woman next to me chose a slice of black forest cake. Her husband glared at her and said, "You're not supposed to have dessert. You know you're watching your weight."

The woman pressed her lips together, set down her fork, and stared at the piece of cake in front of her. Then shrugging, as if to rid herself of her husband's words, she lifted the fork, loaded as much of the cake onto it as possible, and smacked her lips to indicate her enjoyment as she swallowed it down. Glancing in my direction, she said, "He thinks when he talks like that it's for my own good, but it just makes me eat even more."

Immediately, I could relate. Who of us hasn't had the experience of resisting when somebody tells us what to do and claims it's "for our own good"—as if we didn't know? On the other hand, we know the advice is good, so why do we resist? The truth is, most of us don't want or need self-righteous advice from somebody else. And perhaps it's a healthy sign of independence to assert our rights. As an adult I tend to think, "I'll make my own mistakes, thank-you-very-much!"

However, there is another side to this coin. One of the reasons we believe we don't need somebody to tell us what to do is because we have our own built-in critic. But is our own Inner Judge any more helpful at keeping us on track than the self-righteous advisors in our lives?

"Fear of Self-Indulgence" Trap

When Dr. Kelly McGonigal teaches her course on The Science of Willpower, she is often surprised at how fervently her students object to the idea of self-forgiveness, even though it is a proven

WHY OH WHY DID I EAT THE WHOLE CAKE?

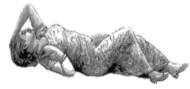

way of increasing willpower. They believe that they must be as self-critical as possible at the first sign of backsliding, or else their dissolute, immoderate, slothful side will overtake them.

Keeping our Inner Dictator primed to make us feel bad when our willpower fails seems the sensible thing to do. We know how easy it is to slide into overindulgent habits, and when all is said and done and the cake is gone, we don't let ourselves off the hook that easily. We assume that only a good mental thrashing will keep us from complete surrender to the lure of our Inner Glutton.

Nevertheless, the evidence is clear that self-criticism is just as *ineffective* at increasing willpower as criticism from others. More self-reproach actually adds up to less motivation and worse self-control. As if that's not bad enough, self-criticism is also one of the biggest predictors of depression.

Are you thoroughly confused now? It's not exactly up-lifting to realize that we rebel, not only, against advice from others, but also against our own good advice. So what's a person to do? Well, most of us look for a reasonable method of dealing with our undesirable behaviors. However, once again, one of the most popular "common-sense" remedies has a built-in trap that captures many of us unawares. See if you can relate.

Escape From "Bad Feelings" Trap

Some people actually do seem to forgive themselves. I often hear people say, "Why should I feel guilty? I refuse to beat myself up." But how exactly do they manage to stave off their bad feelings? Are we to believe that we should eat the whole cake and blithely pat ourselves on the back, too?

Say you're at work and there's a cake for a colleague's birthday. You've been carefully avoiding all "forbidden foods" such as cookies, cakes, pastries, and such. You tell yourself you won't have any cake but when somebody hands you a slice, you feel obligated to eat it. What happens then? Do you tell yourself it's okay? After all, one piece isn't a big deal. Or do you think, "I've blown it now so I might as well have more."

Researchers have documented this common phenomenon in which even one bite of a "forbidden" food can set off a person's belief that they've lost control. This belief is so ingrained that it only takes one cookie or one bite of a fattening food to pave the way to a binge that might last several days before a person regains self-control.

Imagine that in the past you have felt guilty when you give in to these foods and blow your good intentions. But you've now decided you're not going to feel guilty because it doesn't help. So what do you do next? Unfortunately, many people repeat the very thing that made them feel bad in the first place and indulge in yet more of the restricted foods.

Dr. McGonigal has found that one of the main reasons this pattern persists is that it fulfills our need to escape from the bad feelings caused when we lose control. And what is the most expedient means of escape? Why, to have more of the very thing that you were forbidding yourself. After all, consuming the taboo food not only gives the feeling of "self-forgiveness," but it soothes the emotions. It also enables you to avoid the fact that you're right back in the cycle of indulgence.

> **YOU DON'T HAVE TO EAT ALL THE CHOCOLATE TO PROVE THAT YOU'VE LET GO OF GUILT**

On some level, of course, you're aware that you're only putting off the inevitable bad feelings and that they will resurface once the cycle has played itself out. But as long as you keep eating, you can forget about that and indulge in the comfort of those enticing, forbidden foods.

- Do you sometimes feel guilty for eating too much?
- What is your method of escaping from bad feelings?

Getting Beyond The Traps

All the significant battles are waged within the self.
- Sheldon Kropp

If guilt and recriminations don't work, and giving in to more of the same isn't the answer, what is a person to do? How can we forgive ourselves in a way that is helpful, yet avoid being led down the path to more of the same? Well here's some advice from the experts.

What if, instead of listening to criticism, you were to consult a wise, yet compassionate friend? But rather than looking outward for that kindhearted friend, perhaps you would be better off looking inside. Buried beneath the critic who tells you what a wimp you are, and the inner con who goads you on to eat more cake, you discover your true friend. Your very own wise inner advocate.

The truth is, ultimately, you know what's best for you, but it's easy to get bogged down in a rigid struggle between **YOU ARE YOUR OWN WISE ADVOCATE** "good" and "bad." Imagine that you have just fallen off the wagon and eaten that big piece of cake. Your critical side jumps in with words such as: "Now you've done it; you've lost control." For a moment you believe that you have lost control and reach for another piece, but then your inner advocate steps in.

Do you think this compassionate friend will tell you to comfort yourself with the very thing that is creating the problem? Or will she demean you and put you down for having a piece of cake? Not likely. A true friend will help you let go of guilt while still holding yourself accountable for your choices.

Imagine you are listening to your wise advocate—your Inner Guru. You hear comforting words such as, *"Nobody's perfect. Everybody loses control sometimes. This is a human struggle and you can move past this setback."*

Researchers have discovered that no matter how much the notion goes against common-sense belief, the best way to sidestep the out-of-control eating habit is by making effective use of self-forgiveness. This doesn't mean going ahead and eating everything in sight and then feeling happy about it. Self-forgiveness starts with a simple acknowledgement that setbacks are part of life.

Without guilt and the need to escape from it, you can sidestep a further slide into sloth and put your energy and intellect into developing a plan that will enable you to manage your impulsive emotions instead of allowing this side of you to be in control.

What words will your wise inner advocate say in the future to enable you to forgive yourself and move on without sliding into overindulgence?

Stumbling blocks are so plentiful and come in so many forms that it's impossible to cover them all. The next chapter will deal with a few more psychological traps, this time in the form of "good intentions". See if you can relate to any of the following behaviors that most of us fall into with the best of intentions.

CHAPTER 8

"GOOD INTENTION" MYTHS

The road to...extra weight...is paved with good intentions.

Good Intention traps are particularly tricky because they seem to make sense on a rational level whether or not they really do any good. What's more, because good intentions are inspired by positive impulses or, at the very least, harmless intent, we believe that, therefore, they must have a positive effect. And sometimes they do.

The other side, however, is that we are individuals, and each situation takes place within a context. But when good intentions are applied generically, without thought to your own specific needs and tendencies, you could mindlessly be draining your self-esteem by saying or doing things that put a negative spin on your ability.

See if you can relate to any of the following five examples, and if you recognize yourself at all, you just might begin to notice other "obvious" things that you say and do because everybody knows "for a fact" that they are helpful. Sometimes a simple matter of "tweaking" a good intention is all it will take to transform it into a good outcome.

Myth # 1
I'm Investing In Myself

Motivation is what gets you started. Habit is what keeps you going.

-Jim Ryun

I was shopping one day and decided to look in the sporting goods area to see what was new in exercise equipment. Hope lies eternal, and every once in awhile I get this little rush of optimism that I'll see something so profoundly innovative and simple that even I will be motivated enough to use it consistently and really get into shape.

I was perusing the numerous gadgets—big balls, a stepping machine, another device to firm the thighs—but nothing really motivated me. Just then a woman came along and picked up one of the handheld weights. Noticing that it was a heavier size, I thought she must be experienced and might have some advice to fire up my enthusiasm. "Do you do much weightlifting?" I asked.

She looked at me. "I have the lighter ones, so I thought I'd get some heavier ones to go with the set."

"So you really make use of them?" I persisted.

"Not yet," she said. "I haven't used them at all, but I want to." Then she pointed to a large piece of equipment. "I have one of those, but it doesn't do everything that the one at the gym does, so I don't really use it either. I think I need one that has more features."

I looked at the large exercise device and noticed the equally large price tag. "Are you saying you don't use it?"

She shrugged. "Not yet. But I just don't have time to go to the gym, so I'm making my own gym at home. Once I have everything I need then I'll get motivated."

We chatted a bit more. The woman told me that she believed it was important to invest in yourself even if it cost quite a bit. "It's the intention that counts," she said. I didn't reply, but decided to purchase two small, handheld weights. When I departed, the woman was still trying to make up her mind what to buy to add to her growing supply of equipment that—so far—she hadn't used.

We shop for gadgets, devices, and weight-loss products with the best of intentions. But I sometimes wonder what it is we are really shopping for? Is that special piece of equipment going to make the difference?

Or, might it be that we're shopping for something more elusive—that indefinable thing called motivation?

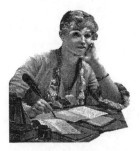

I'VE OVERSPENT ON
MOTIVATION
AGAIN AND I'M
STILL NOT
MOTIVATED

Myth # 2
I Need To Spread the News

I WANT TO ANNOUNCE MY LATEST FAILURE!

One of the things that we often do when we plan to make a change in our lives is to broadcast it. Tell the people we are close to—and maybe even those we aren't. We assume that by talking about our intentions we will have people encouraging us, giving us feedback, helping us along and making sure we follow through.

Telling others is a good common-sense rule of thumb. But sometimes "uncommon" sense is a better strategy. What if we tell everyone our intentions and then fail? Or we don't get around to starting the big diet on Monday. If we lapse, we'll feel all eyes on us every time we bite into something that maybe we shouldn't. It's enough to make a person think twice about even starting a new eating plan.

Most of us have been down the winding road of dieting before. We know what it feels like to face people when the plan flops. As a result, we often put off change, waiting until we are well and truly psyched up before even attempting to begin. Meanwhile, what happens? We're munching away on everything because once all eyes are on us we won't be able to indulge.

In addition, not everybody will be as supportive as we hope. Some of our acquaintances may be so judgmental that we hesitate even to begin. If we fear humiliation, we are less likely to make any change and will continue to wait for sufficient motivation, afraid to expose our weakness by making a half-hearted attempt. So the inner conflict continues. Our rational side doesn't want to be made a fool of and our emotional side doesn't want to be deprived.

That's the beauty of lowering your expectations; you can just go ahead and begin. You don't have to tell anyone. Quietly make a small change that isn't even noticeable. No need to make any announcement. No need to have all eyes on you, watching to see if you are really going to succeed this time.

"But," you ask, "how can I make such a change without being obvious?" Speaking from my own experience, I've found that it's not a big deal to say, "I'll pass on dessert," or even, "I have a bit of indigestion," or "I'll take a piece of cake home for later." If you typically eat fast and have two helpings, then slow down and have one. Nobody will notice—except your waistline. Small changes typically go unnoticed until they add up.

You may find that saving a few calories can be a delicious secret of your own. Your self-confidence will get a boost, too, as you realize you can make a change without making it into a big deal. In time, your secret will speak for itself.

Imagine making a small, yet private, change.

> *No trumpets sound when the important decisions in*
> *our life are made. Destiny is made known silently.*
> **- Agnes Demille**

Myth # 3
I'm Too Old

"How old would you be if you didn't know how old you was?

- Satchel Paige

One of the most frequently cited excuses for weight gain is the age factor. *"The pounds are creeping on because I'm getting older. My body doesn't cooperate anymore. It's not my fault that I'm too old."* Does that sound familiar?

Even today, in our enlightened time, getting older is often equated with a sharp decline in ability. Of course, if you are in poor health you won't feel great, no matter what your age. But many older people are in fine health. Even more are still in good enough shape to enjoy many of the finer things in life.

I believe that each one of us has two ages—one that reflects our chronological clock and another that reflects our quality of life—and they aren't necessarily the same. If we focus on how old we are chronologically, it's easy to fall into a habit of blaming age for every negative thing, including extra weight. But think again! No matter what your age, the power of the "mindless margin" will work every bit as well if you are over sixty-five as for someone twenty years younger, and it takes just as little effort.

Several years ago, my mother, then in her eighties, complained that her clothes were getting tight around her waist. She decided it was just "old age" catching up with her, but grumbled at the thought of buying a larger size. A few months later, she told me something puzzling had happened. "My clothes have gotten loose around my waist. I can't figure out why," she said.

I asked her if she'd been eating differently but she shook her head. "I've been cooking and eating the same as always." Then another thought occurred to her. "A couple months ago I quit taking sugar in my tea," she said. "I usually have dessert so I thought I didn't need the sugar too. Do you think that could be it?"

Clearly, the sugar was it. Yet the change had been small enough that she had to think hard to figure out what she'd done differently. No big lifestyle change. No restrictive diet. Yet the small change was enough to make a significant difference over time. Even at her age.

> "It doesn't happen all at once . . . you become.
> It takes a long time."
> – Margery Williams

Recent statistics indicate that people who reach one hundred represent the fastest growing segment of the population. Yet many people in their fifties and sixties complain that age is their problem. But once again, evidence shows that apart from heredity, what influences us the most in the aging process is our attitude and the choices we make in our activities and the foods we eat.

> *Newly elected President Franklin D. Roosevelt came to call on Justice Oliver Wendell Holmes and asked the older man why he was learning Greek (at his age.) "To improve my mind, young man," was the reply.*

I'm not suggesting that you learn Greek, but keeping mindful of small challenges that take you in a positive direction is the best prescription at any age. And keeping your mind sharp by coming up with small creative strategies is an option without age limit.

> *"If I had known I was going to live this long*
> *I would have taken better care of myself."*
> **– Mickey Mantle**

Myth # 4
But I Have To Lose Weight First

I May Not Be Totally Perfect
But Parts of Me are Excellent
-    **Ashleigh Brilliant**

-

Do you think you have to lose weight before you have the right to look in the mirror and feel good about yourself? Wearing something that you like and that flatters you is one of those little things that can boost your self-image and make you feel like stepping out with confidence. Don't fall for the idea that this is a privilege reserved for the thin (or the rich). An outfit needn't be expensive or extravagant, but a little style can do wonders for your self-esteem. And there's an unexpected ripple effect that might give you an advantage you haven't even considered.

Brian Wansink illustrates this in his book *Mindless Eating: Why We Eat More Than We Think*, when he describes a puzzling pattern of weight gain by inmates at a Midwestern jail. Although the inmates complained about the terrible food, those incarcerated for six months or longer gained an average of twenty pounds. At the same time, they didn't complain about boredom or lack of exercise—the facility had good provisions in those ways.

When the inmates were released and got back their own clothes, they immediately pointed to an unlikely culprit behind their weight gain: the baggy orange jumpsuits they had to wear for the duration of their stay. Without belt notches to signal they were taking in too many calories, their awareness of when they'd had enough to eat was blunted. And they didn't even notice their expanding waistlines because the baggy clothing camouflaged the extra pounds.

Most of us know what it's like when our clothing starts to feel tight. In fact, people report the fit of their clothing as one of the main signals motivating them to cut back on calories. When I read the story of the inmates and their baggy outfits I had to smile, as recent experience made me relate all too well.

I was traveling with a friend for an extended period, and as happens in such cases, we ate many of our meals at restaurants. I suppose I vaguely noticed that some of my clothes were a bit tight, but I thought it was because they had shrunk due to frequent washings. So I decided to buy a couple pairs of loose-fitting pants.

I told myself they were rather stylish and the feeling of pulling in the belt was a bonus. What I liked best of all, however, was that they were comfortable—even when I overate. As time went on and I continued to creatively try new dishes at different restaurants, I was pleased when my pants remained quite baggy. Until I saw a photo of me walking down the street—from behind.

When I saw the photo, I received my wake-up-call. My formerly baggy pants were no longer oversize. Because they were too large to begin with and the belt still had a notch or two to go, I blithely ignored that I was growing into them until I saw the evidence in the photo.

> *This above all: to thine own self be true...*
> **- William Shakespeare**

I took the facts to heart and decided to deal with the setback. Although I continued to frequently eat at restaurants for the duration of the trip, I became mindful of my choices and the amount I consumed. And I went back to wearing clothing that fit well enough to keep me aware of my waistline and make it difficult to ignore the evidence.

That doesn't mean that you should rush out and buy a new wardrobe, but relying on clothing that allows you to expand your comfort level too easily can work against you.

Don't wait until you've lost weight to reward yourself with non-food treats. Little things that make you want to look in the mirror and appreciate the good qualities that you already have can signal a priceless message. The message that you respect yourself and the body you are in—today.

Ashleigh Brilliant makes the point with witty aplomb in his famous quote: *"I may not be totally perfect, but parts of me are excellent."* Focus first on what you like about yourself, then decide on one small step that you can take to build from there.

Myth # 5
Health Foods will Make Me Healthy

The difficulty in life is the choice.
- George Moore

The other day I ran into a friend while shopping for groceries. We were in the cereal aisle and when she saw me, she held out a package. "Look at this," she said. "It's a breakfast bar with fiber and chocolate chips. I need more fiber and I love chocolate. And this is healthy too."

Ever the skeptic, I took the package and turned it over. *Oh-oh.* 14 grams of sugar, plenty of salt, 140 calories. And how much fiber? I was astonished to see that one bar contained a measly 2 grams, a very small amount when you consider that 25 grams is the minimum amount of fiber recommended per day. At the same time, the maximum recommended amount of sugar is 24 to 30 grams. Therefore, one bar would have provided my friend half her daily sugar allotment and less than one tenth the fiber requirement. Yet the label featured "high fiber" but said nothing about the "high sugar".

That encounter made me curious and when I got home, I did a quick search on the Internet where I found a long list of comparisons for cereal bars. I clicked on several and discovered that most had high amounts of sugar—with one exception. The low-carb variety had only a small amount, which perplexed me until I realized the trade-off. The low carbohydrate bars had a lot more fat—saturated fat. In fact, most had twice as much saturated fat as one egg.

Not long before that, I had my own experience in being influenced by advertising when I tried a new yogurt featured as *99 percent fat free*. I was in a hurry and picked up a six-pack carton without reading the ingredients. On the way home in the car I polished off one of the containers. Although I mostly buy plain yogurt and add my own fruit, this one had fruit on the bottom and I was so impressed with the flavor I had a second one when I got home. After all, it was such a small container and, at 99 percent fat free, it had to be healthy. Right?

Several days later when I was down to the last container, I finally took a few minutes to read the ingredients. The first thing I noticed was that the advertising was accurate—barely a trace of fat. Feeling a glow of virtuosity about my good choice, I glanced at the rest of the list and came to a quick stop when I read the words: *27 grams of sugar*. I took another look, not trusting that I had gotten it right. But alas, on second reading I couldn't deny the facts. One small 6 ounce container had more than 5 teaspoons of sugar. No wonder I'd been noticing a decrease in my willpower. On days when I ate two, I was consuming double the maximum daily sugar recommendation in yogurt alone.

So why is it that we consumers are so easily swayed into believing that a food product is healthy because of a few words on the package? Well researchers have that question figured out too. In fact, Brian Wansink uses the term "halo foods" to describe types of foods and wording that many people automatically associate with a health benefit.

For example, when we see phrases such as *low-fat*, *good source of fiber*, or *no trans-fats*, we often conclude that the product is healthy. In addition, foods that fall into the category of yogurt, granola, oat-bran, energy drinks, protein bars (to name a few), trigger a signal to the mindless part of our brains that we are in healthy territory. Moreover, from a psychological point of view, when we believe a food is healthy, we automatically think we can eat more.

My point in telling you this is not to turn you off healthy types of food categories. Fortunately, there are many nutritious choices available—although it can take a bit of searching to find them. The main thing to recognize is that you can easily check out the true health benefit by reading beyond glib advertising and thinking for yourself. Just because a product *doesn't* have a particular unhealthy ingredient, such as saturated fat, make sure you know what it *does* have—then compare the trade-offs.

HALO FOODS MIGHT TRICK YOUR MIND BUT THEY WON'T TRICK YOUR BODY

What many people find helpful is to do a little research, narrow down a few products that meet their requirements, and stick with those. By doing so, you are less likely to be outwitted by advertising gimmicks disguised as health benefits.

I still contend that you *can* have your cake and eat it too. It's good to indulge once in awhile, but at least make an informed choice. Know the difference between good nutrition and dessert. Don't hide your head in the sand when it comes to slick advertising. The "halo food" effect might trick your mind—but it won't trick your body.

Myth # 6
I Deserve A Treat

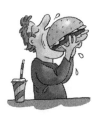

I was having coffee with some friends when a woman I'd only met once before, let's call her Kathleen, joined us. She'd just come from the gym and was annoyed to discover that she'd gained five pounds since starting her exercise program. "They promised me I'd lose weight on this program and the opposite has happened. I feel like demanding my money back," she said, then turned to the waiter and ordered a specialty coffee with whipped cream and a scone with cream cheese and preserves. "I'm always so hungry after these workouts," she continued. "But after all that work and sweating I figure I deserve a treat. I must have burned off more than enough calories."

FOOD FOR THOUGHT

- 30 minutes of swimming laps burns 300 calories
- One small pack of peanuts has 300 calories
- There are 500 calories in a large muffin

When we think of exercise solely in terms of weight loss, we are more likely to give it up when the pounds don't melt off. But because our bodies conserve energy, it takes a lot of exercise to burn a significant number of calories. A half hour of intense aerobics or swimming, for example, will only burn between 200 and 300 calories. Kathleen's specialty coffee alone had cancelled out the weight-loss benefits of her workout, and the scone added a few hundred extra.

Does that mean those of us who are not into vigorous exercise should just give it up as having no benefit? Well, as it turns out, this is another case where the obvious isn't as it appears. When it comes to exercise there is a secret value that many people are not aware of.

> *Beware lest you lose the substance by*
> *grasping at the shadow."*
> **- Aesop, Aesop's Fables**

So read on to discover the true benefit of exercise—the hidden bonus that goes beyond weight loss yet still provides the boost to help you reach your goal. And don't fear. Even the lazy types who cringe at the thought of strenuous exercise can reap the rewards. I will attest to that.

Myth # 7
I'm Waiting for a Magic Remedy

Some women ask the question, "Isn't there a pill, or something quick and easy, that will melt away the fat? I just want to it to be gone." Well, I do know that there have been many attempts at coming up with an effortless remedy such as a pill, but to my knowledge, none, so far, have been truly successful.

Even if you could eat whatever you wanted and then take a pill to keep you thin, you might be thin but you would likely also be sick and miserable and foggy minded. How appealing is that?

But guess what? Researchers have established the one thing that is as close to "magic" as anything is so far. No, it's not in the form of a pill and it does take a bit of exertion. But the output of energy is minimal, not overly demanding, and only takes a small amount of time. You already know what it is, but in keeping with an open-mind policy, read what the experts have to say about an old form of "magic" with a bit of a different twist.

Researchers Megan Oaten, a psychologist, and Ken Chang, a biologist, at the Macquarie University in Sydney, Australia found that exercise can give you a huge advantage in every area of your life, as well as making your weight management endeavors more successful.

I know, I said I don't go in for much exercise. However, I do believe in incorporating physical activity into my daily routine, even if it doesn't look like exercise. Here are the benefits their research findings turned up:

- Willpower benefits of exercise are immediate
- Only fifteen minutes on a treadmill reduces cravings
- Even small amounts of exercise help to reduce stress
- Over time, exercise is as powerful an antidepressant as Prozac
- Exercise increases the baseline heart variability and trains the brain

Notice that the above benefits do not require you to leap into an organized exercise program. Even fifteen minutes of consistent activity can lower stress and boost your will-power.

And take note of the fact that weight loss is conspicuously absent from the above list. Yet the number-one reason that people embark on an exercise program is because they believe it will make them lose weight.

Thinking mindfully of the advantages of exercise *beyond weight loss* will protect you from walking into the trap of starting a program and then giving up altogether if you don't see a quick weight loss. Once again, raising awareness and recognizing the true benefits of consistent activity will give you a big advantage in many ways.

Small steps add up and, in the big picture, exercise will help your body become more efficient at burning calories too. That means your "willing" biology will be more willing to let go of those additional pounds. By all means— replenish your energy with food—but pause and think before you choose.

JUST 15 MINUTES MAKES ME FEEL SO MUCH BETTER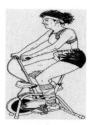

- Have you ever dropped out of an exercise program because you haven't lost weight?
- Think of 3 ways that you can incorporate 15 minutes of consistent activity into your daily routine.
- Now choose one.

CHAPTER 9

FOOD TRAPS

Genetics Versus Biology

In their fascinating book *Food Fight: The Inside Story of The Food Industry, America's Obesity Crisis, and What We Can Do About It,* Kelly Brownell, and Katherine Horgen explore the popular debate: What is the cause of obesity? Genetics or environment? They explain that while it takes a "willing" biology to gain enough weight to become obese, it's the environment that causes it to occur.

> "Genes load the gun, the environment pulls the trigger."
> - Obesity expert: George Bray

If you are one of the unfortunate who easily gain weight, you're not alone. A recent statistic on this category stated the number of people in the obese bracket to be over four billion in North America alone. A mind-boggling number that makes it clear: *Many, many people have a "willing" biology when it comes to gaining weight.*

A prime factor in this conundrum, is that foods high in calories and fat have become extremely convenient and a common part of our daily consumption. What's more, because our genetic ancestors have not always had a continuous supply of food, our bodies were designed to store fat in times of plenty to prepare for lean times ahead. But in today's society most of us don't experience those lean times, which makes our modern-day environment ideal for creating exactly the problem we see—a nation of overweight people.

Unfortunately, our inner calculator does not instinctively send out signals when we've had enough. I know—it doesn't seem fair that we should be designed to want to eat all that we can without an internal switch that will automatically kick in when we've had enough. Which means we're stuck with a love-hate relationship with food—we love to eat all those goodies—but we hate feeling stuffed or sick.

The fact that you're reading this book means that you're likely trying to figure out how to regulate your food intake. But avoiding foods that deplete, rather than replenish, your physical and mental needs can seem as confusing as putting together a thousand piece puzzle of a blue sky. However, a little "food" education can go a long way, and once you become more aware of the numerous ways that you get trapped by food, you'll develop an ability to come up with strategies to help you take intelligent control of your food choices.

When Are You Full?

How do you know when you're full? Do you stop half-way through a meal and consult your stomach? Or do you keep eating until you've finished what's on your plate? Most people aim to finish what's in front of them before consulting with their stomach and asking whether it is full enough.

But does your stomach tell the truth? Say you're at a family dinner or a buffet, and you eat until you're so stuffed that you can't swallow

> *"It is a hard matter, my fellow citizens, to argue with the belly, since it has no ears."*
> **– Plutarch circa 45 – 125 A.D.**

another bite. Until dessert is served, and magically your stomach makes more room. How does this happen? Surprisingly enough, researchers have found that the stomach has only three main settings when determining how much is enough:

- Starving
- I'm full but I can eat more
- I'm stuffed

Dr. Barbara Rolls of the Center for Behavioral Nutrition at Penn State has conducted thousands of hours of lab studies which confirm that unless we're stuffed or starving, we really don't know when we've had enough to eat. This is good news, because with a little planning we can redesign some of our eating habits to save on calories yet still satisfy our desire to feel full. What it takes is a strategic method to satisfy our hunger on different levels and thus outwit our less than accurate hunger gauge.

As we've learned, we're creatures of habit. So in order to eat less and still feel satisfied, we need to fulfill our feeling of what is "enough," rather than trusting our stomach to tell us. One key factor that we can use to our advantage is that we eat with our eyes, and when our eyes see something that isn't the usual size, our stomach gets the message.

Say you're used to a burger that's big enough to hold in two hands. You know from experience that it will fill you up. But you're trying to cut back on calories, so you go with the smaller burger. It arrives with a skinny slab of meat and cheese between a bun, and you can pick it up in one hand. What happens? Very likely your eyes will say that it's not going to fill you up. And chances are they'll be right. Even though you might save 500 calories, you're not likely to feel satisfied and might be tempted to order something else, hardly a satisfactory outcome.

Dr. Rolls found that if a person who is used to eating a half-pound hamburger is served a quarter-pounder "dressed up" with extra lettuce and tomato instead, it will appear similar enough not to be obvious. They'll still feel full.

Research has repeatedly proven that appearance wins 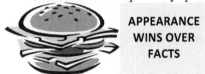 **APPEARANCE WINS OVER FACTS** over the facts: if it looks large and we think the portion will make us full, we'll feel satisfied and save hundreds of calories. What a creative way to outwit your unreliable hunger gauge and save and shave calories while still enjoying tasty, nourishing foods.

Warehouse Shopping Trap

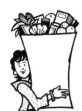

Food psychologist Brian Wansink points out that the supersize superstores are not always such a bargain. He calls this the "warehouse club curse" because of the traps built into shopping in large quantities. Say you buy a value-size carton containing 36 packs of bite-size cookies (100 calories a pack). A good way to limit those calories, right? You're putting away the groceries and decide to have one pack—a mere 100 calories—and you gobble them down in a few bites. Then you look at the carton, which has 35 more packages. Compared to all those packages the one that you ate seems like nothing. So you have another, and then maybe another after that.

Because our eyes rather than our stomachs tell us when we've had enough, we compare what we've eaten with what's still left. When we see so much, our "stop" signal grows weaker. Rationally, we know the idea behind 100-calorie packs is to have only one, yet it's too easy to ignore this fact. Have you done this? If so, you've been caught in a trap. It's obvious—in fact you sort of know it's there—but you walk into it anyway.

Another warehouse trap that Wansink points out is the "cabinet castaways" syndrome. Although we eat more when there's abundance, this tendency only lasts for the first week or so. Then some of the products become "cabinet castaways," ending up at the back of the shelf or falling to the bottom of the freezer. When it comes time to clean out the freezer and the kitchen storage areas, many of these products get thrown out. There goes the extra value.

That doesn't mean wholesale clubs are never a good deal, but we should only load up on what we really need. If I buy ten pounds of onions for nearly the same price as five pounds or five pounds of carrots for only a bit more than the two-pound bag, or get a large sack of apples on sale, that's value.

But buying the enormous container of ice cream is a different matter. I have no problem resisting the lure of onions, carrots, and even apples as I silently beat a path past the pantry, straight to the freezer and the bargain size container of cookie dough ice cream.

Economy-Size Containers

One day while shopping for groceries, I decided I wanted a sweet treat and headed for the cookie aisle. After studying several shelves with every imaginable type of cookie, I realized they all had one thing in common. They came in large packages. I wanted a treat—not a pig-out—and I knew I couldn't trust myself with a monster bag of chocolate chip cookies, so decided on a second choice. A single chocolate bar.

The snack aisle also had an array of choices, but I soon found my favorite. When I picked it up, however, I saw that it, too, had miraculously become larger—one third larger, as the packaging announced. I experienced a moment of elation as my emotional side perked up at the prospect of more chocolate. But I also realized that the new, larger size also contained a third more calories. Exactly what I wanted to avoid.

So, in addition to the added temptations of "big value" packaging, I discovered that it's difficult to find snacks in the old-fashioned regular size. This means that if we want to outwit our desire to eat more, we have to become even more creative.

Over and over, researchers have found that when we dig into a large bag of chips, cookies, or anything else that's sweet or salty, we consume more. Remember, stomachs don't count calories, and we can consume approximately twenty percent more or twenty percent less without even being aware of it.

It used to be that special treats came in one-serving packages, making it far easier to eat just that amount. Now we are faced with the choice of either trusting our future self to have more self-control than in the past—or coming up with alternatives. Here are a couple of ideas to get you thinking:

- Food experts advise measuring single-serving amounts into smaller-portion bags. When you reach into the cupboard for a snack, it will already be prepackaged and you won't have to rely on your eyes or your stomach to tell you when you've had enough.
- Instead of buying a bag of cookies or a whole cake, go to a bakery and buy single-size servings. It costs a bit more, but in the end you save calories—and maybe even the cost of those "cabinet castaways."

Booby-Traps

> *THE BEST PLACE TO HIDE ANYTHING IS*
> *WHERE EVERYONE CAN SEE IT.*
> *-SHERLOCK HOLMES*

The dictionary defines a "booby trap" as a device designed to capture the unwary. Such traps are also sometimes used to trick the unsuspecting as a joke, which gives them an impression of innocence. But when it comes to food-related booby traps, these devious little tricksters catch us all the time. Because of their sheer abundance and the fact that they blend in with our surroundings, they are particularly difficult to identify as a problem. In fact, we sometimes rig our own booby traps.

Researchers have come up with the top five places where such traps are commonly found:

- Home
- Office
- Grocery stores
- Restaurants
- Kitchen

Do you keep a bowl of candies on your coffee table or your desk at work? Who would suspect that an innocent bowl of candy could have any real effect on weight? However, Brian Wansink discovered that candy bowls can be subtle little culprits. They catch people exactly because they appear so harmless. And not all candy bowls are created equal.

In his study, all the secretaries in a large office building were given a covered dish of candy to be kept on their desk. Half of the dishes were clear so the candies showed through, and the other half were white, so with the lid on the candies were not visible. Every night when the secretaries went home, the researchers counted how many candies had been eaten, then replenished the dish. Two weeks later they compiled the results. Secretaries given the clear see-through dishes ate 71 percent more candies than the secretaries with the white covered dish. That's 77 more calories a day.

The point of this research was to study the effect of visible foods versus foods that are out of sight. The food experts found that this effect follows us throughout the day. We eat more of visible foods because the sight of something tempting requires us to draw on our willpower reserves to resist it.

If the temptation happens to be in the form of a clear candy bowl on your desk, you might be saying "no" every five minutes—every time you turn your head. That's a lot of pressure on your willpower muscle. Eventually you're bound to give in and say "yes," as attested by the secretaries.

Other studies confirm this effect. Out of sight, out of mind—but the more we see of tempting foods, the more we eat. The visibility trap can add unwanted pounds; the 77 extra calories a day consumed by the secretaries add up to five pounds of weight a year.

Fortunately, researchers also provide ways to counter the visibility traps, although it can take some concerted effort. For example, when healthy foods are out in the open, we tend to eat more of them, too. By replacing a cookie jar on the counter or that candy bowl on your desk with a bowl of fruit, you are more likely to eat a healthy snack without even thinking about the pack of chocolate candies that are out of sight. Yet another trick is to organize the eye-level shelves of your cupboards with the healthful snacks in front, where you'll see them whenever you open the cupboard.

Another influential booby trap appears when we have to contend with the power of association. If walking past a bakery or driving past a fast food outlet fuels an irresistible invitation to go inside, why not take a different route? Avoidance is often the most practical way to keep from overstressing and depleting your willpower reserves. Going a few blocks out of your way might save you a lot of empty calories and conserve your energy to discover new and better choices.

The Convenience Trap

How Far will you go for a chocolate? When a temptation is convenient, we're more likely to give in. Say you have a box of chocolates in your refrigerator. You're sitting on the sofa watching television and you think of the chocolates. What are the chances that you'll get up at the next commercial and go and get the chocolates? But what if you had to get dressed and go to the store for chocolate? You're far more likely to resist that inconvenient temptation.

CAN YOU RESIST YOUR FAVORITE TREAT WHEN IT'S RIGHT IN YOUR KITCHEN?

Even rats will eat more when food is convenient. In a lab experiment, rats had to press a lever ten times to get food pellets. Apparently, ten times isn't too much for a rat, so they ate regularly. But when they had to press the lever 100 times, they made do with less food.

Once you start noticing the convenience and visibility traps that litter your environment, you can take measures to clear as many as possible. Don't make it easy to have what you know you shouldn't.

At a time when I particularly wanted to avoid such foods, I received a box of chocolates. I knew that if they remained in my kitchen, the lure of those chocolates would get to me. My condo was on the tenth floor of a high-rise, and, as it was winter I decided to put the chocolates into the trunk of my car. The strategy worked. When I thought of the chocolates, I also had to think of whether I wanted to go downstairs to the chilly parking area to get one. Like the rats, I ate the inconvenient treats less often.

The mind is endlessly creative when it wants to get something that you don't need. Make that creativity work in your favor by coming up with ways to defeat the booby traps in your life.

Hidden Calorie Trap

The hidden calorie trap is another way that extra weight catches us unawares. Because hidden calories don't look like a piece of chocolate or a peanut, we often don't have any idea of the quantity we are consuming. Fortunately, sharpening your awareness can save you calories without causing you to feel deprived.

One food that often comes disguised as a low-calorie choice is salad. People order salad as a healthy way to increase fiber and decrease calories, then they cancel out the benefits by pouring on the dressing and other popular top-pings such as cheese flakes and bacon bits. What starts out as a potentially healthy choice becomes a high-calorie, high-sodium trap.

Sandwiches can be another food trap, especially if they come from a restaurant or food chain. For example, one popular food chain advertises a chicken salad sandwich as "all white meat." Surely chicken breast must be a low-fat choice. Yet the sandwich has over 1000 calories. How can that be? Well guess what. It's not the chicken, it's the dressing.

Food chains compete for customers, and to make sure the patrons keep coming back, they devise ways to make their special sandwich extra tasty. Unfortunately, the wonderful taste that keeps you coming back is the high-fat, high-sodium dressing. Researchers found that many of these seemingly innocent sandwiches can run between 1000 and 1700 calories, more than half a day's worth of calories for most women.

The "Crispy, Battered Nugget" Trap

Don't dig your grave with a knife and fork.
                        - English proverb

Anything "crispy" or "battered" announces another fat trap. You might think that a crispy chicken breast or battered fish sandwich is a relatively good choice, but even if there is nothing but air inside the tasty exterior you will be consuming high calories, sodium, and fat. Not a good combination for keeping your mental and emotional motor running at optimal level, let alone your weight.

That doesn't mean there aren't low-calorie, low-fat options on many restaurant menus. However, when researching the viability of low calorie alternatives, food experts made an interesting observation. Restaurants that offer low-fat choices do attract more customers, but once inside, the vast majority of people end up ordering the high-calorie fare. Apparently, just thinking about choosing a healthier item makes people feel better about themselves, so when they go ahead and choose the high fat items, they wind up with less guilt.

Maintain a measure of skepticism when something you think of as *healthy* is also deluxe, crispy, or shaped like a nugget. Do yourself a favor by choosing foods that will sharpen your mental and emotional capacity and keep you looking and feeling great throughout the day.

CHAPTER 10

THE FOOD THERAPY ADVANTAGE

Food is an important part of a balanced diet.
— Fran Liebowitz

Timing: When You Eat and What

Do you follow the nutritional food guidelines and eat three balanced meals a day? Not too long ago, people routinely ate breakfast, packed a lunch for noon, and sat down to an evening meal. Today the three-meal-a-day rule simply doesn't fit most people's lifestyle.

It's not uncommon to pull into a fast food restaurant for a take-out meal or to pick up something from the deli on the way home. As for breakfast, that could be a muffin and coffee on the way to work. And what about packing a lunch? Almost unheard of.

As a result, we have far less control of, or information about, the quality of foods we consume, and when the weight starts piling on we often don't know where it's coming from. Because food is so emotionally charged, when we don't have guidelines that are easy for our rational side to enforce, our inner con moves in to take charge of those choices. That means the burger and fries will win out over a sensible meal unless you come up with a workable strategy. Workable: that is the key.

I have found that a helpful way to raise awareness and promote conscious eating is to loosely structure food choices into categories rather than rigidly designating meals as the dividing line. These boundaries are not brick walls, but once you see and feel the benefits of choosing foods from within certain guidelines, selecting better choices becomes less of a chore for your rational side.

Because food choices have a real impact on your quality of life, not just in the future but on a day-to-day basis, learning to consciously choose the foods with the biggest payout and smallest hardship is one of the most important skills you can master.

"Live happily ever-after—one day at a time."

Over the years, I've learned to choose foods that will optimize my daily quality of life. The method that woks best for me is to categorize my food choices based on physical, mental, and emotional needs, choosing the foods that match whichever of these needs I am trying to fulfill at the moment. Of course, most of life is fairly routine, and my schedule is quite ordinary. Most of us tend to have times when we want to maximize energy and alertness, usually during work hours. At other times, we want to enhance relaxation. And let's not to forget the times when we look forward to special events—and perhaps more indulgence.

These boundaries are natural, and therefore it pays to become keenly aware of how best to feed your body in order to satisfy your current need. For example, if you choose the same type of food when you need to be mentally alert as you do when you want to relax in front of the TV, you could end up eating more of what your body doesn't need without feeling satisfied, and in the process wind up consuming a lot of empty calories.

This doesn't mean I deprive myself by refusing to enjoy the full range of foods; rather, I enjoy them more because I'm eating what I need when I need it. The following chapters will explain this concept in more detail, but for now, here are the categories that seem to encompass most food choices:

1. Fuel food
2. Savoring food
3. Snacking food
4. Luxury food

Fuel Food

My favorite animal is steak.
— **Fran Lebowitz**

Does it seem strange to think of food as fuel? I started thinking this way after a learning experience that occurred during a period in my life when I made frequent long road trips. Sometimes, I would be on the road all day, and therefore my requirements for staying alert were particularly important. But even though I made a point of getting a good sleep the night before, I'd still get extremely fatigued over the course of the day.

I didn't look forward to these long trips, but I had an established routine that at least gave me something to anticipate. Every time I stopped to fuel my car, I'd get some "fuel" for myself, too. I would drive for a couple of hours, then stop and pick up a coffee along with an oversized muffin that I slathered with butter. My lunch stop consisted of a burger and fries with more coffee. By mid-afternoon, I really needed an energy boost and would usually get an ice cream cone and stock up on a chocolate bar or two to keep me going during the final leg of my trip.

Topping up my "fuel" with sweets as a way to replenish my energy seemed like a good idea, as I'd read that sugar gives a quick energy boost. Yet often my energy became so depleted that the chocolate bar would only sustain me for a short while. Eating another one didn't help, either.

This was also the phase in my life when I started making conscious changes in my eating habits. One of these changes was to pack a lunch for work instead of eating deli foods during the day. So, on my next road trip I automatically packed some food to take along, thinking that I'd save some calories this way. Just as bad habits have a way of spreading and permeating many areas of a person's life, so do good ones.

Instead of the big muffin, my first stop consisted of coffee with whole grain toast and a boiled egg. I didn't want to cut out all of my treats because that was part of the anticipation of the journey, but instead of a burger and fries I ordered only the fries to eat after my tuna sandwich. That way I satisfied my emotional side but still kept my calorie intake down. I still had an ice cream cone sometimes, but cut out the chocolate bars altogether.

By making those few simple changes in my usual road-food choices, I was able to fuel my energy requirements each time I stopped to put gas in my car and still cut down on calories without feeling deprived. To my surprise, I also noticed an unexpected benefit that was perhaps even more important than the calorie savings. A benefit that made me realize yet another unexpected advantage of making conscious food choices.

The Energy-Mood Advantage

I only get grouchy and moody on days that end with Y.
                                        - Anonymous

Remember, the change in my food choices were motivated by a desire to manage my weight without restrictive dieting. However, it took a couple more road trips before I noticed a pattern emerge. I would arrive at my destination feeling reasonably energetic instead of burned out and irritable. That was a surprise since I'd come to accept the burned-out feeling as a normal side effect of a long trip. What's more, I didn't need a sugar fix to get me through the last leg of the journey as I had in the past.

When I finally made the connection between the change in my eating habits and my energy level, it was another one of those "ah-ha" moments. Once again, I had caught myself doing something right.

As mentioned in an earlier chapter, when researchers tested people who were glucose deprived they discovered that low glucose translates into low self-control. And according to nutritionists, the best way to maintain a steady supply of the type of glucose that doesn't cause the crash-and-burn cycle, is to choose low-glycemic foods. Foods such as lean proteins, high-fiber grains, fruits and vegetables, and nuts and beans. Exactly the type of food I had chosen to "fuel up" on my trip.

One of the more important messages I took from that experience is the value of "fuel food" during times that require both mental and physical energy. This type of food is not meant to stimulate the taste buds but to burn slowly, thereby giving your body a consistent level of energy while preventing the mood swings that are associated with dips in blood sugar. For me, daytime hours are when I usually need to remain alert and focused to help me be more productive. Therefore, I make a conscious choice NOT to graze on the "treat" type of foods that I am likely to eat when I'm socializing or relaxing. As a result, I look forward to snacks and specialty foods with more anticipation. The payoff is a healthier, trimmer body, a clearer mind and fewer mood swings.

> **FUEL FOODS KEEP YOU MORE ALERT AND AWARE WITHOUT OVER-STIMULATING YOUR TASTE-BUDS**

Here are some of the foods I have found to work best for me during the times when I need more energy. In making my choices, I look for foods that are fairly light in calories, nutritious, and boring enough that they don't get me obsessing about food, yet are also energizing and satisfying.

- Eggs (poached, omelet or boiled)
- Whole grain bread
- Fruit (apple, orange, berries or other fruit in season)
- Fish (any fresh fish is excellent, but salmon is particularly healthy and filling)
- Chicken
- Beef, lamb, pork (a good way to eat the leftovers)
- Tuna, salmon, sardines (tin)
- Vegetables (crunchy such as cauliflower, broccoli, carrots, etc.)
- Cottage cheese (zero or 1% fat)
- Milk (skim or 1%)
- Yogurt (low fat without sugar—add your own fruit)
- Beans (such as garbanzo, kidney, black beans, etc)
- Quinoa (a grain-like seed high in protein with all nine essential amino acids)

Use your creativity to make fuel foods more appetizing. For example, you can make a dip from beans to go with your crunchy veggies, but watch out for the crackers. Also, if you like yogurt, some of the new Greek varieties have double the protein. However, beware of added sugar. A much better option is to add your own fruit to yogurt or add yogurt to soup or creamy sauces for a rich, tangy flavor.

A recent study revealed that one of the reasons that diets work is because they limit variety, which makes them "boring". As a result, dieters are less likely to want more of the same. So why not harness the "power of boredom" when you are eating for energy by choosing foods that motivate your vitality instead of your taste buds!

Savoring Food

Eat less, taste more."
- Traditional Chinese proverb

Typically, evening is the time associated with slower dining and relaxation. A time that many of us anticipate after a day of work or other activity. And that's good; anticipation is a powerful motivator. Yet if you eat consciously during the day, then go home and have pizza, chicken wings, or other quick foods as your evening meal, on a regular basis, you will lose the benefits of your daytime mindful choices.

What works best for me is to make my evening meal moderately special, different from my daytime eating style. I want it to be tasty and well balanced but not overly fancy or time-consuming to prepare.

Food researchers and nutritionists recommend the "half-plate" rule, which is to fill half of your dinner plate with vegetables and the other half with protein and starchy food. As much as I try to eat vegetables during the day, I fall short on that one. So I make a point of including some crunchy vegetables such as broccoli or cauliflower in a salad or lightly steamed, or perhaps green or yellow beans as part of my evening meal.

But what if you don't cook? What if you're perfectly happy with a steady diet of fast food for your evening choice? After all, isn't pizza supposed to be good for you?

If your food style includes an abundance of fast foods, here's some information to take into consideration. While some fast foods are clearly a better choice than others, you still need to be careful.

More than one study has revealed that when food is chemically changed to appeal to our taste buds without satisfying our nutritional needs, it can become insidiously addictive—much like an addictive drug. When rats were fed a steady diet of fast foods then switched to healthy foods, they refused to eat—even to the point of near starvation.

Hopefully, we humans are smarter than rats, but many people do consume a steady diet of fast foods and don't want anything else. If you are trying to counter that trap, remember the wisdom of "living in the moment".

Challenge yourself to come up with creative ways to transform your evening food experience into a relaxing and enjoyable process that will support—instead of diminish—your quality of life. For example, listening to music and sipping a cup of tea or a glass of wine can enhance the task of chopping vegetables.

After all, how much time and effort does it really take to put a portion of chicken with some veggies and potatoes into the oven? Only a few minutes—then you're free to kick back and relax or do whatever your schedule requires and smell...not the roses...but the comforting aroma of real home-cooking. Whether you are preparing a meal for a table of one or for a larger family, you can keep your choices simple and nutritious and make the process something to anticipate.

> *Health is not simply the absence of sickness.*
> **- Hanna Green**

If you persist, your body will adjust and automatically crave what's good for you. Once this happens, your will-power muscle will be energized instead of exhausted. Then the struggle between the rational and emotional will calm down and, at least for a while, your two sides will be on the same side—craving the benefits of better health and well-being.

My usual standbys for evening meals are:

- Chicken
- Lean Beef
- Fish
- Lamb
- Lean pork
- Legumes (black beans, lentils, etc.)
- Raw vegetables
- Steamed vegetables
- Stir-fried veggies

- Salad (be careful of heavy dressings)
- Soup
- Potatoes
- Whole-wheat pasta
- Brown rice

Remember that natural spices are a great way to enhance food flavor. Savory spices tend to signal your brain when you've had enough, unlike fatty, high-salt, and sweet sauces, all of which over stimulate the taste buds, making it more difficult for your body to register the signal "I'm full enough".

Snacking Food

No man in the world has more courage than the man
who can stop after eating one peanut.
~Channing Pollock

Looking back, I can see how naive I was when I started my quest for weight management without dieting. When I first realized that I had cut out evening snacking because of my busy schedule, I thought I'd found the answer. All I had to do was say "no" to snacking in the evening. The premise worked—as long as my schedule kept me too busy to think about snacking.

Once I finished my coursework, however, I once again had more leisure time in the evenings. Unfortunately for me, relaxing entertainment triggers the need to find something to munch on. Every time I turned on the television or picked up a magazine, I wanted a snack. Clearly "just say no" didn't work when my elephant-sized emotions were stirred back to action. Yet due to my limited experience, my rational side had been lulled into the belief that my snacking problem was under control.

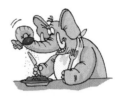

I DEMAND MY SNACK NOW!

Now I know better. I still struggle with the urge to eat more sweets and snacks than I would like, but I have come to expect this and prudently developed strategies for dealing with my cravings. Back then, however, I was taken by surprise when I realized I had not "cured" myself of snacking. Which left me with two options: Either outwit my emotional hankering to nibble on sweet, fatty, rich snacks in the evenings, or, get ready to go shopping for a larger sized wardrobe.

I did manage to find several low-calorie snacking foods such as yogurt and fruit, but I missed my unhealthy treats and craved something crunchy (other than raw carrots). The reality, however, is that peanuts, corn chips, potato chips, cheese twists, and what-have-you, are all loaded with calories. Really loaded—unless you stick to a handful. For me, a handful was not—and still isn't—a satisfying snack.

This was back in the days before microwaves and all the 100-calorie snack packs that flood the market today. My options seemed extremely narrow, but based on the positive experiences I'd had when I opened my mind to possibilities, I decided to approach the challenge with an open mind.

And Then I Found It...

> *Always approach a case with an*
> *absolutely blank mind, which is*
> *always an advantage.*
> **– Sherlock Holmes**

I was browsing in a shop one day—not thinking at all about what would help my snacking situation—when I spotted my solution on a shelf. At the time, it was a rather new contraption—a hot-air popcorn popper. I always associate popcorn with good times from my childhood and the hot-air popper promised to produce a large bowl in a few minutes without any oil or added calories. Talk about good news! To me it seemed the ideal answer.

Some people consider hot-air popcorn to be boring. But it is the one most amazing thing that saved me from snacking my way back into a larger size. The trick with this type of popcorn is to eat it while it's warm. I drizzle on some light butter or light margarine and salt. As well, a simple internet search will provide a variety of ways to jazz up the flavor. It's crunchy and tasty, and a big bowl will fill you up without triggering your taste buds into an all-out gorge.

When I still want something sweet as well, I've found that hot chocolate (light) or flavored low fat yogurt is a great combination. Pairing the popcorn with fruit works well, too, as taken together they satisfy the desire for something crunchy, salty, and sweet all in one sitting.

By substituting hot-air popcorn for more high-calorie food, I found a way to trick my taste buds and calm my emotional side when it demanded a crunchy-salty snack. Of course, this strategy doesn't work all the time but, even so, every time it does, you gain an advantage. Try it. You just might get to like it, especially if you can find creative ways to dress up the popcorn without adding too many extra calories. Beware, however. Not all popcorn is created equal.

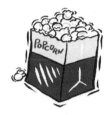
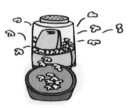

**THEATRE POPCORN
CAN BE MORE
THAN 700 CALORIES**

**3 CUPS OF HOT AIR
POPCORN IS LESS
THAN 100 CALORIES**

Movie popcorn is loaded with enough calories and salt to put anyone over their limit. And researchers have discovered that salty foods can increase your craving for sweets. Even relatively healthy snacking foods tend to be high in calories and salt. For example 1/3 cup of peanuts or trail mix contain over 300 calorie. And that's only enough to get most of us started.

On the other hand, a cup of light hot chocolate with a big bowl of crunchy, hot-air popcorn gives a lot more value for the calories and provides a portion that will satisfy most appetites. Doesn't that make more sense?

Luxury Food

"Extravagant and self-indulgent" are words the dictionary uses to describe luxury. Who doesn't want a little self-indulgence once in awhile?

ENHANCE YOUR EATING PLEASURE BY ANTICIPATING SPECIAL FOOD OCCASIONS

What makes luxury food special, however, is that this type of food is not meant to be an everyday event. Even a culinary extravaganza loses its special status if you have it too often. And that quality of "specialness" is one of the most enticing things about luxury foods and food-related events. Anticipation is half of the enjoyment.

When you make your list of luxury foods, pay attention to the frequency with which you consume them. Many people can, and do, have luxury foods on a daily basis, but in doing so they diminish the pleasure of the experience.

Here are a few of my luxury foods. You will notice that some items are far from "luxury" in terms of our cultural habits, but even something like a chocolate bar is special for me because I don't have one every day. As a result, I enjoy it even more when I do, plus I feel more positive about taking control of food choices knowing that I am not consuming too much sugar and high fat on a daily basis.

Some of My "Luxuries"

- Dining out—grilled steak, pasta with sauce, seafood in cream sauce, ribs
- Fast foods—pizza, burgers, fries, deli sandwiches
- Sausages, bacon and prepared meats
- Special desserts—cake, ice cream,
- Specialty drinks—Frappuccino, hot chocolate with whipped cream, milkshakes
- Cocktails
- Special snacks—chocolate bar, chips, dip, cheese and crackers, nuts, cheese twists, etc.
- Sweet or heavy dressings, sauces and dips

When you keep rich, sweet and fatty foods in the special "luxury" category, you do your body a favor. Not only are you cutting back calories, but with better health and energy, you increase your quality of life. There is a time and a place for everything and that includes a time to enjoy what is truly "special."

To be without some of the things you want
is an indispensable part of happiness.
- **Bertrand Russell**

Keep Your Perspective

My food categories are not rigidly fixed, but on a day-to-day basis, I've come to see the importance of having a plan that I can count on that satisfies my energy needs and also takes into account my basic desire to snack and munch. If you can stop after a small amount of high-calorie snacks, you don't need to be concerned about the snacking trap. But if one bite of something sweet or highly salty often gets you eating too much, then you need to be honest with yourself and come up with a backup plan for your every-day treats.

Remember, there are *no* forbidden foods. However, I've come to the conclusion that timing is one of the most overlooked, yet important ingredients when formulating a personal food plan.

By maintaining awareness of your needs at any given time—whether a high-energy output time or a time of relaxation—you will enhance your quality (and possibly your quantity) of life, by keeping food in its proper place.

CHAPTER 11

End Notes & Reminders

It is good to have an end to journey toward;
but it is the journey that matters, in the end.
— Ursula K. Le Guin

R emember, there is not one fixed answer for everybody. Therefore, you need to maintain your toolkit of strategies and ideas so you can continue to renew and spark your creative side. When you have only one tool—such as dieting—as your mainstay to keep your weight under control, you are far more likely to keep repeating the same experience with the same result.

Following are the highlights of the concepts that are covered in the book. Use them as quick reminders to help you stay on path. Bon Voyage and Bon appétit.

OPEN YOUR MIND TO POSSIBILITIES:
- Encourage an open mind policy
- Notice the times when you are eating better.
- Take on a detective persona
- Observe and reflect on new information
- Keep a journal of important points

UNCOMMON-SENSE CONCEPTS:
- Never underestimate the power of your emotions
- Don't get stuck in blaming the past
- Use past information to recognize patterns
- Do more of what's working
- Lower your expectations
- Appreciate the satisfaction of "good enough".
- Prepare for failure and setbacks.
- Expect fear
- Face fear straight on

OUTWIT RESISTANCE:
- Remember, everybody resists change
- Recognize your obstacles
- Use baby steps to overcome resistance
- Boost your staying power with small rewards
- Satisfy your emotional side to ease the process

ILLUMINATE YOUR JOURNEY
* Focus on the process rather than the result.
* Luxuriate in the journey to better eating habits
* Notice small positive changes
* Do more of what works

CHECK YOUR MINDSET.
* Embrace a "learner" style
* Recognize the value of Effort and Persistence
* Choose an "open-mindset."
* Accept that setbacks are part of life
* Persistence wins over natural-born talent.

ASSESS INCOMING DATA
* Habits are necessary for survival
* All habits are stored in your mindless data base
* Beware of mindless food choices
* Diminish the power of bad habits by increasing good habits

UNDERSTAND THE MEANING OF WILLPOWER
* Willpower is similar to a muscle.
* Don't over-stress your willpower muscle
* Eliminate unnecessary temptation
* Build strength-of-will by saying *No* to small urges
* Identify Willpower Traps to conserve your energy
* When in doubt, consult your *Wise Inner Advocate*
* You must *eat* to resist overeating—choose wisely

BEWARE OF GOOD INTENTIONS
- Recognize that the best of intentions can backfire.
- Be alert to mindless choices
- Question the status quo and try something different
- Monitor your thinking habits
- Be aware of "halo" food traps
- Take a minute and read the ingredients
- Recognize the value of exercise beyond weight loss

RECOGNIZE FOOD TRAPS
- Be mindful of the peril of big bargain shopping
- Distinguish between quality and quantity
- Beware of Booby-traps in familiar settings
- Recognize hidden calories in "innocent" foods
- Don't make it easy to have foods you don't need
- "Houseclean" food traps to cut down on temptation

APPLY THE FOOD THERAPY ADVANTAGE
- Evaluate what you eat and when you eat it.
- Make use of "Timing" to increase quality of life
- Maximize your energy by choosing fuel foods
- Enhance eating pleasure by keeping special foods "special"
- Embrace the power of "boring" foods to energize your body without stimulating your taste buds
- Determine whether you are eating for power, pleasure or leisure
- Pinpoint your needs when making food choices

ABOVE ALL, START SMALL...BUT START TODAY
AND BE KIND TO YOURSELF

RECOMMENDED READING

I would highly recommend any of the books that appear in the reference list. However, the following I have found to be particularly helpful for those struggling with food habits:

The Power of Habit: Why We Do What We Do in Life and Business by Charles Duhigg

One Small Step Can Change Your Life—The Kaizen Way by Robert Maurer Ph.D.

The Willpower Instinct: How Self-Control Works, Why it Matters, and What You Can Do to Get More of It by Kelly McGonigal Ph.D.

The Volumetrics Eating Plan: Techniques and Recipes for Feeling Full on Fewer Calories by Barbara Rolls Ph.D.

Mindless Eating: Why We Eat More Than We Think. By Brian Wansink

References

Baumeister, R.F. and Tierney, J. (2011) Willpower: Rediscovering Our Greatest Strength. New York: Penguin

Brownell, K. and Horgen, K.B. (2004) Food Fight: The Inside Story of The Food Industry, America's Obesity Crisis, and What We Can Do About It. New York: The McGraw-Hill Companies, Inc.

Conan Doyle, A. (1998) The Complete Sherlock Holmes: All 4 Novels and 56 Short Stories: Bantam Doubleday

Dweck, C. (2006) Mindset: The New Psychology of Success. New York: Random House

Duhigg, C. (2012)The Power of Habit: Why We Do What We Do in Life and Business. New York: Random House

Haidt, J. (2006) The Happiness Hypothesis: Finding Truth in Ancient Wisdom. New York: Basic Books

Heath, C. and Heath, D. (2010) Switch: How to Change Things When Change is Hard: New York: Random House

Maurer, R. (2004) One Small Step Can Change Your Life – The Kaizen Way. New York: Workman Publishing

McGonigal, K. (2012) The Willpower Instinct: How Self-Control Works, why it matters, and what you can do to get more of it. New York: Avery

Polivy, J. and Herman, P. (2002) If At First You Don't Succeed: False Hopes of Self-Change. American Psychologist

References

Rolls, B. and Barnett, R.A. (2000) Volumetrics: Feel Full on Fewer Calories. New York: Harper Collins

Seligman, M.E. (1991) Learned Optimism: How to Change Your Mind and Your Life. New York: Knopf

Wansink, B. (2006) Mindless Eating – Why We Eat More Than We Think. New York: Bantam Books

P.S.

If you have any questions or comments, please feel free to contact the author at: Fridaypublishing@gmail.com.

If you would like to leave a short review or comments regarding the book, you can do so on the Food Therapy book site at Amazon.com or Amazon.ca.

—————Marlene Laszlo

About the Author

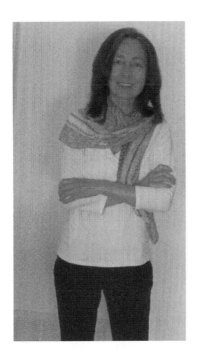

Marlene Laszlo is a seeker of possibilities, an author and, most importantly, a gatherer of food-related information. Her work as a psychotherapist introduced her to solution-oriented concepts that she applied in her own personal struggle with weight. People often tell her that she is "lucky" because she can eat whatever she wants. But the truth is, weight management has little to do with "luck".

Food Therapy is a combination of her personal experience, solution-oriented concepts, and strategies and research findings to support her method of conscious eating.

13454631R00075

Made in the USA
Middletown, DE
17 November 2018